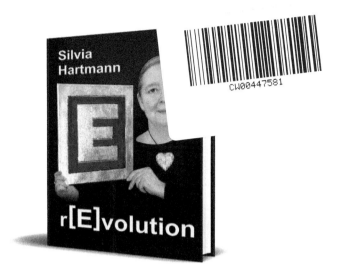

The Modern Energy

rEvolution

Silvia Hartmann

Published By

The Guild of Energists

www.GoE.ac

Love this? Join the GoE, take courses and talk to the community:

GoE.ac/Join

The Energy rEvolution
Silvia Hartmann
1st Print Edition 2023
ISBN: 9781873483138
Published by DragonRising Publishing for The Guild of Energists GoE.ac

By This Author:

EMO Energy In Motion
Modern Energy Tapping
Infinite Creativity
Star Matrix
The Power Of The Positives

Table of Contents

Foreword To The 3rd Edition by Silvia Hartmann

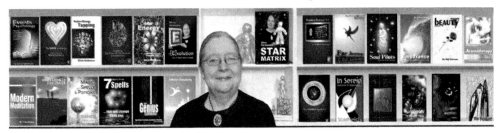

I have a very important question for you.

"What is the most important part of you
that receives the least amount of attention?"

Well, that would be your living energy body.

Your own, real living energy body which contains that heart that can break, produces all of your emotions, and your personal key to immortality, the immortal soul.

You might think that this extraordinary third component in the mind, body, SPIRIT (energy body) triad would receive our interest, our preferential focus of attention and all the care we could possibly give it – but nothing could be further from the truth.

The current paradigm in the western World, and all who look to the western World for guidance and leadership, is locked in a vicious circle stemming from a reality divergent paradigm - the mind/body duality.

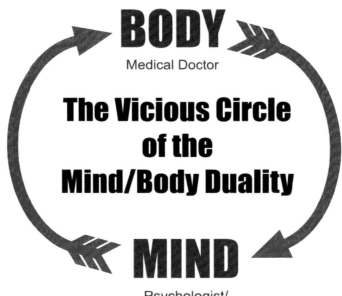

BODY

Medical Doctor

The Vicious Circle of the Mind/Body Duality

MIND

Psychologist/
Psychiatrist

The "mind/body duality" is a perfect example of a reality divergence – operating on a model of reality that is faulty in some way. In this case, here is a reality reduced model that is missing 33.3~% of actual reality by completely ignoring the third part in the mind/body/SPIRIT aka ENERGY BODY **triad.**

This missing information causes all manner of chaos in the systems built upon such a faulty model, and the problems created in this system cannot be resolved from within it.

For example, as much as 50% of people presenting to medical doctors with physical symptoms receive the diagnosis "No medical cause." They are then referred to the "It's all in your MIND department," but that doesn't cure their symptoms, so they go back to the medical doctor for more tests. Each time a person goes around this loop, they become more distressed, and their symptoms are getting worse.

This vicious cycle is also in operation the other way around, where a patient may present with a variety of problems which are diagnosed as "mental problems," but when a mental solution cannot be found, then a medical solution is being applied and chemicals that cause physical reactions in the physical body are prescribed. These do not cure the problems either, and round and round we go.

The fundamental problem we are dealing with here is not that individual medical doctors and psychologists/psychiatrists are not sincerely trying to help the patients; the fundamental problem is the mind/body duality paradigm.

When we add the third point, the missing Third Field, we make a true paradigm shift into a better model that is closer to reality absolute, answers so many questions that could never be answered under the old paradigm, and makes many more questions entirely irrelevant.

Most importantly, by adding the Third Field to the fundamental care of the citizens, we are no longer stuck and brand new ways, ideas, research directions present themselves and evolution can finally occur.

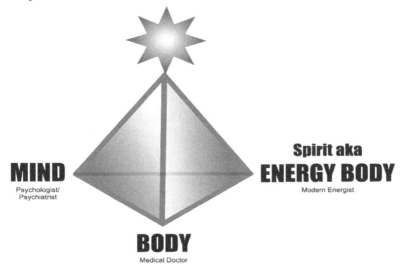

As I write this, the chances of any established institutions built on the mind/body duality paradigm adopting this more reality based view of caring for the mental, physical and emotional well being of its citizens adopting this paradigm shift are infinitesimally small.

However, someone has to start somewhere, and this is what I and my fellow Modern Energists are dedicated to.

With the many financial benefits involved in sending citizens around in an endless loop between mind and body only, from which there is no escape, creating the "eternal patient," Modern Energy has to be a grass roots movement.

This means that one individual at a time has the chance to think about themselves in a new way; that one person at a time tries out the theory and practice of Modern Energy for themselves, and makes up their own minds whether this is valuable to them at the personal level.

There will come a time when enough single people who understand the truth about energy, about their own living (neglected, forgotten, ignored, disrespected, mistreated) energy bodies come together, and changes will be made.

We absolutely need the Third Field in the mind/body/SPIRIT triad to begin.

We need the new "Science of Love." We need to bring love and logic back onto the same page to start making sense of ourselves, of why people do the things they do, to end an ocean of entirely unnecessary suffering as soon as possible, and to make human being HAPPIER.

This is my wish and my goal, my life's work and why I created the Guild of Energists, The GoE.

I want a rEvolution!

In the following pages, I will share the fundamental principles of Modern Energy.

These did not come from a burning bush, and they were not found in some ancient manuscript in a crumbling temple in a far away land.

Everything you will read in this book was discovered, one step at a time, over the last 30 years, in direct practice with real people from all walks of life, all ages, and all around the world.

I thank you for your time and attention and I hope you will find something in these pages that will inspire you and help you on your way.

With all my love,

Silvia Hartmann

President, The Guild of Energists, August 2022

References:

1. *The Third Field https://goe.ac/the_third_field.htm*

2. *Diagnosis: No Medical Cause https://goe.ac/diagnosis-no-medical-cause.htm*

3. *The New Science Of Love: https://goe.ac/we_dont_need_a_new_religion_we_need_the_science_of_love.htm*

The Modern Energy rEvolution

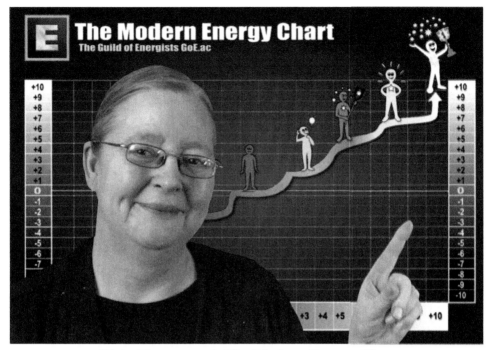

Silvia Hartmann & The Modern Energy Chart

Modern Energy comes directly from a breakthrough piece of research into animal behaviour conducted by Silvia Hartmann in the United Kingdom between 1987 to 1993 which revealed the predictable effects of energy exchanges between social mammals on behaviour.

Silvia Hartmann and her team discovered that energy is absolutely real, that energy states affect performance, behaviour and emotions in the most fundamental way that is easily measurable, and simply structural to social mammals, including human beings.

The Modern Energy Chart was created, and has since been refined over the last 25 years based on the experiences of innumerable people from all walks of life, of all ages, and from anywhere in the world.

From the Modern Energy Chart, new techniques, methods and approaches arise naturally which are likewise clean, logical and precisely predictable in their functioning. We may not be able to see or measure energy exchanges directly, but we can measure their effects.

Modern Energy is not related to or based upon any ancient approaches to dealing with the invisible realities that are nonetheless quite real.

Modern Energy opens up a different world where love and logic are on the same page.

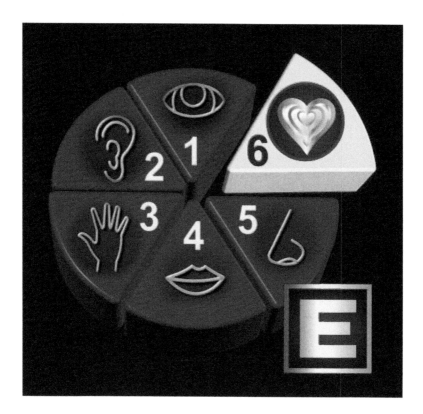

A true paradigm shift occurs when we consider reality with six senses, rather than just five.

Adding that missing 16.7% of information from the 6th Sense changes the world.

⭐ **The 6th Sense is to sense energy, to feel emotions.**

⭐ **Our emotions are our real 6th Sense.**

Emotions are not in the mind or in the head, they are physical sensations that are the feedback mechanism about the state and condition of the energy body.

⭐ **Emotions inform us about what we cannot see, feel, hear, scent or taste.**

Emotions are the key to all human activities. Without understanding emotions, we cannot understand ourselves, each other, or make sense, literally, of the problems that have bedevilled mankind since the dawn of time.

We cannot find solutions to humanity's problems without understanding what emotions are, where they come from, how they affect us in mind, body and spirit.

We cannot evaluate the accuracy of research, theory and science, philosophy and the most essential rules and regulations created by human beings without factoring in which emotional states they came from.

When we do understand what emotions are, literally everything changes.

There is an extraordinary explosion of possibilities, new research directions, a bright and brilliant stream of new ideas and solutions that have never been discovered before.

Modern Energy holds the key to not only our personal evolution, but also to societal and global evolution of mankind.

Here are the basic principles of Modern Energy in a nutshell.

A Super Short Introduction To Modern Energy

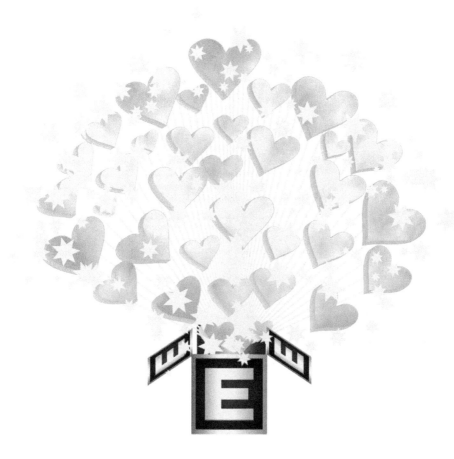

"There is only energy, and the absence of energy."

Silvia Hartmann

The Living Energy Body

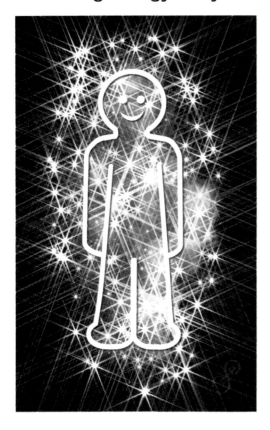

Every person has a real energy body, whether they know this or not.

The energy body transmits its states of being through the medium of EMOTIONS.

Emotions range from fine sensations, also known as intuition, through all the various manifestations of emotions all the way to the high end emotions, known as psychosomatic emotions, which are indistinguishable from physical pain.

- ✖ Modern Energy does not concern itself with physical problems.

- ✖ Modern Energy does not concern itself with psychological problems.

♥ Modern Energy only concerns itself with the energy body.

At first glance, this may not seem as important as physical or psychological problems.

However, there are many problems that cannot be solved in any other way than by treating the energy body, and this of course means addressing the "emotional problems."

Many more problems have an energy component which can influence the severity of the problems.

For optimal functioning, the living energy body is of the essence because is the source of our personal power, and without it, we can't find or understand happiness, can't understand ourselves or other people, can't make sense of the world and certainly can never find enlightenment.

Overall, the living energy body is the structural "back bone" of the human systems of mind, body and spirit.

Our living Energy Bodies are the true source of our personal power.

A strong Energy Body is the basis for a happy, successful life.

The 6th Sense

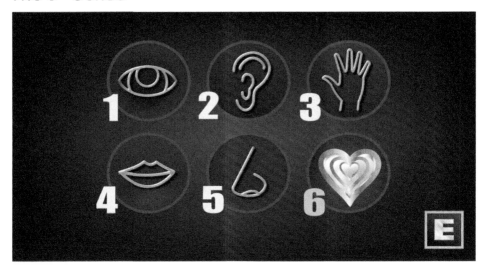

Our true 6th Sense are our emotions.

* Emotions are feedback from the energy body through the physical body.

* The energy body creates sensations that have no physical origin.

* Our emotional state tells us how our energy body is doing.

* **We have the 6th Sense of emotions to inform us about a bandwidth of reality that we cannot see, hear, feel, taste or scent.**

* When we consciously become aware of the additional information from the 6th Sense, we are said to have become enlightened.

When we are happy, in love, feel strong and capable, our energy body is doing well. A lot of energy flows in, through and out the energy body, keeping it fresh and constantly energized.

When we are scared, upset, feel powerless and depressed, our energy body is not doing well. Energy is too low, and we have no energy to deal with life.

People did not understand the connection between emotions and the energy body, and did not give any attention to the many "cries for help" the stressed energy body produces all the time.

Likewise, without even having a concept of the living Energy Body, there could never be a sensible explanation of how people fall in love, how they are inspired, and why some people are successful, when others simply aren't.

Modern Energy focuses on the energy body exclusively, because we now know that when we pay attention to the energy body, not only do our emotions change instantly, but we can also think much more clearly and our bodies become stronger at the same time.

By finally paying attention to our living energy body, we instantly gain a simple, direct path to feeling better, thinking better, acting better and becoming stronger, more successful and healthier.

The Energy Body Stress Factor

Everyone talks about stress, and everyone knows that when you get stressed, you start doing, feeling and thinking things you would never be doing, feeling or thinking on a "good day."

Nobody knows what stress really is however, or how to avoid stress, remove stress, or how to turn stress into success instead.

- **This is because the reality of the living energy body is the missing X-factor in the equation.**

Through sheer ignorance and systemic neglect, modern people's energy bodies are in a state of advanced scurvy.

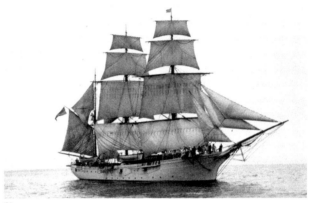

The Scurvy Story

A long time ago, when the first great ships sailed across the oceans of the world, the sailors were beset by many mysterious illnesses.

Their hair and teeth fell out, their bones became weak, their eyesight would deteriorate, their skin would become irritated yet would not heal. The sailors also experienced becoming clumsy and prone to mistakes, falling off the rigging and having more accidents. They couldn't sleep at night and would start to hallucinate and show all the signs of insanity.

The doctors of the time treated each problem separately with all manner of pills, potions and tinctures, but nothing worked – until one doctor finally had the brilliant idea that it wasn't the presence of all these different illnesses that was the problem here, but in fact the absence of fresh fruit in their diet.

Just a few drops of lime juice, and all the many horrendous symptoms went away.

Rather than all these separate diseases, it was <u>the absence</u> of Vitamin C which was destroying the sailor's minds, bodies and spirits.

The energy bodies of modern humans are living in chronic scurvy conditions.

Nobody understand the crucial importance of our living energy bodies, nobody pays attention to their many screams and cries of joy and pain, no-one takes care of them. Our energy bodies are not being fed with the kind of energies the energy body needs to become strong and healthy, to function normally.

There is no pill or potion that can alleviate energy body stress and you can't cure it with material wealth, no matter how many billions you might throw at it. We cannot even know what the real energy problems are whilst they are in such poor condition after a lifetime of neglect, mistreatment, starvation and malnutrition.

⭐ **Above all else, we need to start to feed our energy bodies right.**

We need to give our energy bodies the energy nutrition they crave – the energy vitamins of powerful, positive energies. As soon as we do that, the many symptoms of energy body stress start to disappear, and a different person emerges - someone who is stronger, heals faster, who is more powerful, smarter, and most of all, *happier.*

The Modern Energy Chart

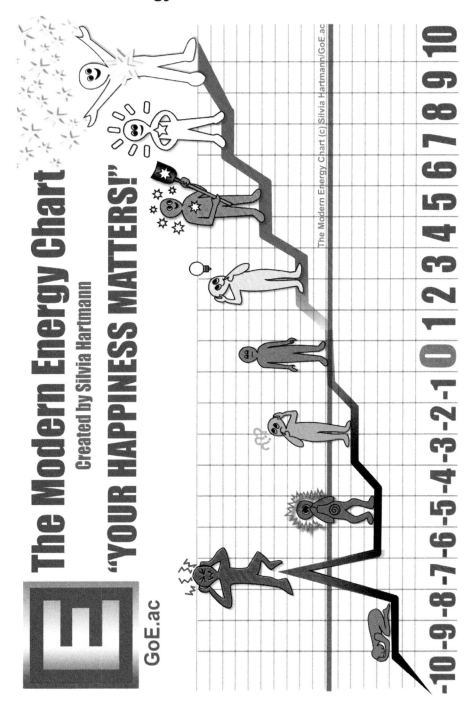

The Energy rEvolution

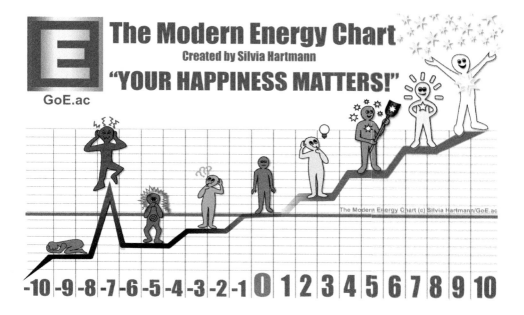

The Modern Energy Chart

Created by Silvia Hartmann

"YOUR HAPPINESS MATTERS!"

GoE.ac

The Modern Energy Chart (c) Silvia Hartmann/GoE.ac

-10 -9 -8 -7 -6 -5 -4 -3 -2 -1 0 1 2 3 4 5 6 7 8 9 10

The Modern Energy Chart shows what happens to a person when their energy levels change.

- Different energy levels in the energy body create different energy states.

- These different energy states create significant changes in mind, body and emotions.

The Energy Chart shows us that any person becomes "a better version of themselves" when their energy flow improves. This improvement is measurable in mental performance, physical performance, social performance and in emotional stability.

- **Any human being at all, regardless how old, young, what their gender may be, their previous experiences or current level of health, will improve when energy flow is increased.**

- **Conversely, any human being becomes less and less effective when the energy body is stressed.**

This has very powerful repercussions for a person's self concept. It finally explains how someone can be sequentially nice and nasty, friendly and antisocial, intelligent and stupid, capable and useless.

- ☆ **How well we succeed at anything at all is dependent on our energy states.**

To understand this also transforms how we understand other people, and how we deal with them. To understand that a stressed person is just stressed (rather than "mad, bad and dangerous" or "born bad") allows us to treat them differently, to use very different strategies to help them and bring them back to better states of functioning in mind, body and spirit.

This is of the utmost importance in dealing with children but also with adults, both in private contexts as well as in professional and business relationships.

- **For personal development and understanding yourself and other people, the Energy Chart is the key to your evolution.**

The Modern Energy Chart In Brief

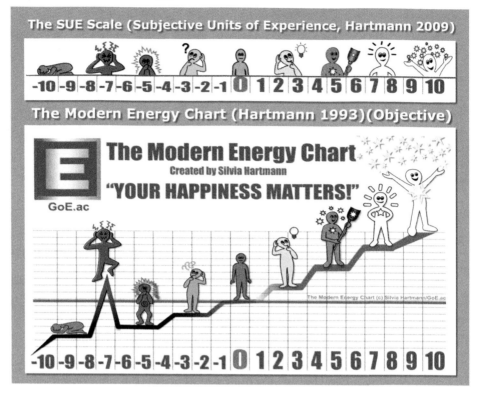

We can measure our energy body states and those of other people using the Modern Energy Chart.

This gives us not only important information about the person, but also the direction in which we want to move if we want this person to be more powerful, active, intelligent, capable, physically co-ordinated and emotionally resilient.

We move upward on the Energy Chart

when we <u>add more energy</u> to the energy body.

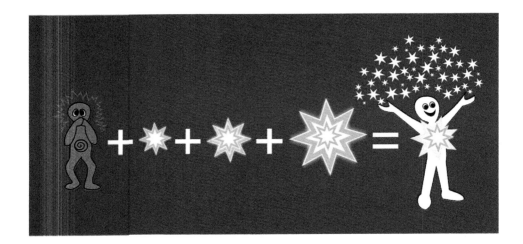

Print out the Modern Energy Chart and hang it on your fridge so that all members of your household can see it, every day. This will help everyone understand how human stress works, and everyone can then work together to help each other become stressed less often.

We can also activate our natural intelligence to find ways to avoid old stress traps, and discover more ways to make ourselves and each other happier.

Once we understand how our energy bodies express themselves through our emotions, we can begin to understand why our happiness is so important – which is why we say:

Your Happiness MATTERS!

Here are the major energy body states in brief.

-9 = The Extremely Low Energy States

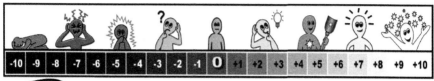

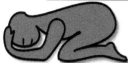

- -8 to -10 describes the extremely low energy states that can become life threatening.

- It takes seriously destructive energy events for energy bodies to become so critically low on energy that they literally collapse in on themselves.

- This can be observed in the natural dying process of old people, but also in people following extreme emotional disturbances.

- At -8, we find all the symptoms previously associated with severe depression. The person at -8 literally has no energy to help themselves or perform even routine physical functions.

- A person at -9 is withdrawn, incapable of making connections with others, incapable of communicating and indeed, struggling to survive at all.

- Depending on the circumstances, people will recover slowly as the energy system strives to repair itself, but if the damage is too severe, the person might never fully recover.

- -10, the complete extinction of the energy body, leads to physical death shortly after. This is the mechanism by which people die of a broken heart.

-7 = The Emergency State

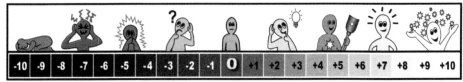

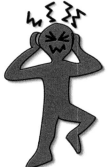

🔴 When energy flow has become critical, an emergency response is triggered in the energy system which will throw the last remaining reserves of energy into the system as a survival effort.

🔴 The affected person will explode into rage or other uncontrollable emotions such as having a panic attack, throw themselves around in a "nervous breakdown" or may attack bystanders randomly.

🔴 There is an explosion of energy at -7 which has confused people for a long time.

🔴 The emergency generator is not a high energy state, it is a critical survival emergency state that should not be used unless it is really a life or death situation, as we would find in the final struggle of a prey animal caught in the teeth of a predator.

🔴 This dangerous energy state is called "Rage Syndrome" in animals.

🔴 In humans, the absence of coherent, logical thought, any understanding of moral values or long term consequences of actions in this state makes it particularly dangerous.

🔴 Further, there will be an energy collapse after the emergency system has been triggered, into the extreme low energy states, and the health of the energy body may be permanently jeopardized.

-5 = Fear

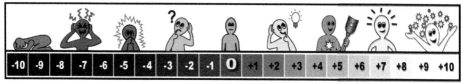

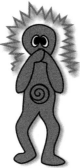

- Around -5 we find high stress, anxiety and fear.

- This denotes an extremely de-stabilised energy body that is on the verge of flipping into the -7 emergency state, where all emotional control is lost.

- The person at -5 and -6 will be incapable of controlling their thoughts or directing their attention.

- They will be paranoid, fearful, startle easily and find it impossible to concentrate.

- They have lost their ability to function correctly in social relationships.

- Their mental abilities and faculties of reasoning are strongly impaired, which can lead to very bad decisions.

- They will typically experience strong 6th Sense sensations, such as shaking, trembling, stomach churning, back aches, headaches etc.

- Their physical performance will be strongly impaired, making it much more likely that accidents will occur.

- When the 6th Sense sensations become overwhelming, individuals might turn to self mutilation to override the psychosomatic pain from their emotions.

-3 = Stress

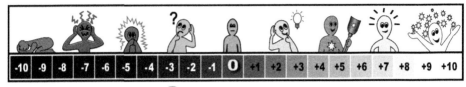

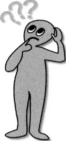

● Uncertainty is the big keyword for the energy body states between -2 and -4. This is where the vast majority of the modern population exists.

● Feeling unsure, unbalanced, not quite right, being easily distracted and not feeling entirely at home in one's own physical body are among the many negative side effects.

● Social functioning and communications are strongly impaired.

● Self doubt is a constant feature of this state.

● A person at this level will feel the need to "follow a stronger energy system" and/or turn to external authorities for guidance and leadership.

● This is a chronic stress state that relies on applying will power the whole time to create a false outward appearance of functionality and achievement.

● Under the old systems which did not factor in the states of the energy body, these stress states were deemed to produce maximum effort from the stressed people involved and were mistaken for "good stress."

● On the Modern Energy Chart, this is a dangerous energy body stress state which will produce inferior performance across the board in mind, body and spirit.

0 = The Zero Point Of Nothing

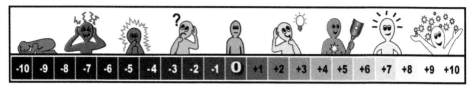

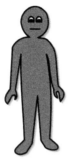

- Having ZERO emotions, feeling nothing at all, feeling neither good nor bad, is the deluded and entirely erroneous goal of the old schools of emotional suppression and mismanagement.

- ZERO is not a place of balance. When you have zero money in your account, zero food in your fridge and zero friends in your address book, this is what you have – ZERO. Nothing. Nada. Zilch.

- Likewise, we also have ZERO intelligence and ZERO logic in this place that doesn't understand people, doesn't understand emotions, and produces truly inhumane systems that will destroy the people who pass through them.

- Getting beyond the Zero Point of Nothing, explaining to people that this isn't good enough, it's NOTHING, actually, is the great challenge of Modern Energy.

- Yes, it is bad to suffer from negative emotions.

- **Having no emotions is not the cure for the human condition.**

- We need to move forward, into the higher energy states and the realms of positive emotions.

+3 = Awakening

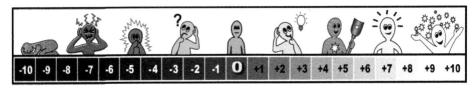

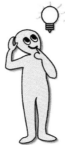

- When energy flow finally improves beyond Zero, and the energy body wakes up, so does the person whose energy body this is.

- Now, a person may have some ideas about the future, might want to improve something, make positive changes, start a project.

- It is important to note that at the low positive ranges, there is enough energy to think, dream and talk about projects, but not enough energy to actually enact them through ongoing, daily, reliable physical labour and high energy activity.

- At the social level, a person's social capabilities increase at +3 and they become more attractive to others.

- They also become more open-minded, mentally flexible, and able to learn more easily as well as remember better.

- As they are now energy positive, they have energy left to give to others.

- This is a good first step towards real energy body health which we find not at +3, but at +10 instead.

+5 = Inspired Action

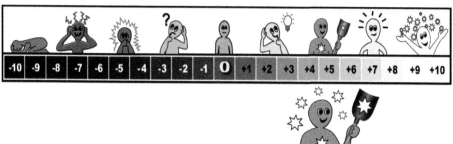

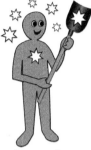

- When the energy body gets to +5, we have the energy to take ACTION.

- To make anything happen in the real world, we need to put in our ENERGY: effort, labour, physical activity, and we have to keep it up on a regular basis.

- Many people have good ideas, but to turn these ideas into something real takes a lot of energy, every single day, and the next day, and the day after that.

- There will be set backs of course that will drop us down the Energy Chart and we might get angry, stressed, afraid or depressed for a while; but we can bring up our energy average back to above +5 so we can take the action we need to take in the real world in order to succeed.

- A very common problem is seen when people have good ideas, are inspired, get started, but then something bad happens and they drop down the energy chart. With energy being now too low to do the work that needs to be done, the project must fail.

- Serial failures in everything from learning via relationships and business success come from this cycle, which we can finally both understand, as well as break, with Modern Energy knowledge.

+7 = Success

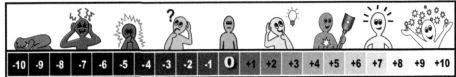

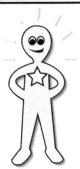

⌣ The previous stage, +5, is the set up for success.

⌣ Working with lots of energy on something we are excited about, not giving up when there are set backs, having good relationships with others and fully engaging with our projects will lead to success.

⌣ Success is a new level of accomplishment and achievement, and it brings many further rewards.

⌣ It raises self esteem, and also allows a person to do energising things, and enrich themselves with objects, activities, environments and people that can further raise their energy.

⌣ A +7 person becomes a natural leader **as people will follow those with higher energy states than themselves**, and gather a high energy team about them.

⌣ From the earthly standpoint, +7 is as good as it gets.

⌣ The person has good relationships, is successful, financially abundant, has many friends and to all intents and purposes, is a role model for success.

+10 = Freedom

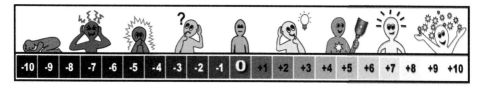

⭐ There is a tremendous threshold shift from +7 to +10.

⭐ At +10, the energy body fires on all cylinders and this brings a tremendous increase in emotional, physical and mental health.

⭐ For as long as human beings have been around, these states were deemed to be incredibly rare, and people who obtained them by accident or incident were thought to be prophets, saints, geniuses, or otherwise blessed by the stars.

⭐ Often, they would bring back a single good idea from these high energy states, where true organic intelligence and real logic are accessible, where cause-and-effect become apparent, where the nature of reality itself becomes revealed to a human being.

⭐ Many times, these people would start a revolution, or a religion, or became famous leaders, artists and scientists revered across the ages.

⭐ **The extraordinary truth is that all normal human beings attain +10 states, that everyone has experienced them already.**

⭐ Not only that, +10 states are easy to achieve once we know that we are simply dealing with the living energy body.

⭐ All we have to do is to feed our energy body, and the +10 experiences cease to be a rare event, and instead, become the structural solutions to our individual problems, and those of the human race as well.

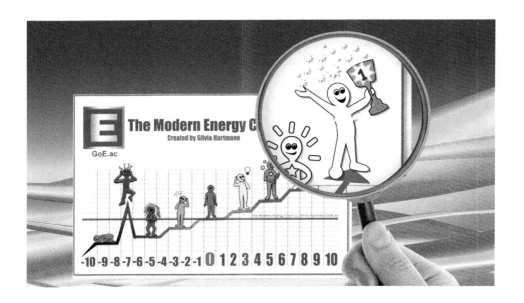

To experience MORE +10 events
is the goal in Modern Energy.

Living Life With A Full Battery

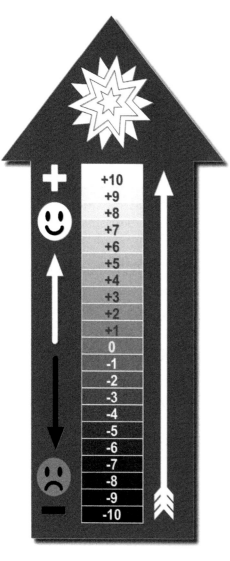

There are all sorts of things modern human beings do which disturb the energy system.

The more stressed the energy system becomes, the worse we feel about ourselves, about other people, about the whole world.

Life becomes hard and painful.

It gets worse as energy flow becomes more and more disrupted.

Low energy flow leads to disturbed emotions, disturbed thinking and makes the body weak as well.

When energy flow is low, we try to live life with a depleted battery.

There is no energy for self healing, never mind self improvement.

We simply don't have the strength to do the work we need to do and we don't have much left to give to others.

We need to learn to quite literally re-charge the batteries of our energy systems - and to do that, we need positive energy that empower the energy system and bring it back to life.

Positive energy feeds the energy body and re-charges your batteries of life.

The SUE Scale

Subjective Units of Experience, Hartmann 2009

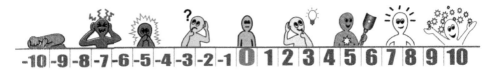

The SUE Scale (Subjective Units of Experience, Hartmann 2009) is the short version of the Modern Energy Chart.

We can ask ourselves and others where they are on the SUE Scale between -10 and +10 at any given moment to make an easy assessment of our energy body states.

Try it now by running your finger along the chart to find the SUE Number that matches your mood in this moment.

- **Moving up on the SUE Scale is the purpose of all Modern Energy systems, methods and techniques.**

For example, we might ask what kind of positive energy would provide a boost, right here and now, to make us feel better.

Learning to take notice of our energy states first of all, and then to take action to raise energy is life changing. Everything we do works better, is easier and more likely to be successful if we are higher on the SUE Scale.

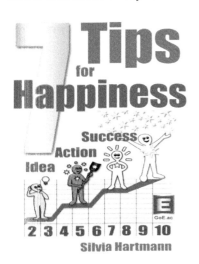

Likewise, starting to look at other people and their behaviours with the SUE Scale in mind will lead to many insights and much, much better understanding of "why people do the things they do."

All Modern Energy techniques and methods are designed to create a movement up the SUE Scale to empower people, quite literally.

- *You can find our favourite simple methods for raising energy in 7 Tips For Happiness, FREE here: https://goe.ac/7tips*

High Energy Flow Is The Goal!

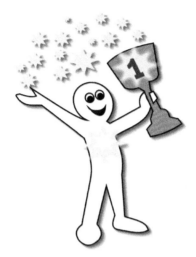

- Our energy bodies works best for us when they are in full flow,

- Full flow means being above +7 on the Energy Chart.

- This is a state similar to when you are in love.

- Gravity is lighter, the colours are brighter, you feel strong, young, powerful and happy in every fibre of your being, wide awake, and you are kind to everyone.

To move into these high energy states,
we need more POSITIVE energy.

- Positive energy lifts our state (of mind, body and spirit!) higher and make us feel glad to be alive.

- We become more powerful, but most importantly, more joyful.

- This gives us real strength and the energy we need to face adversity in life.

- High energy flow gives us the power we need to live rich and meaningful lives.

- **The more we have, the more we have to give!**

Many Different People: The Aspects Model

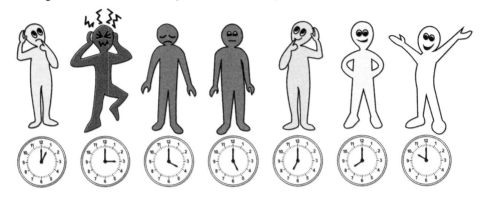

Understanding energy body stress transforms the way we understand ourselves as well as other people.

Every person is many different people - depending on how stressed they are at the time.

To help us understand how this works, we have The Aspects Model in Modern Energy theory.

☆ **An aspect is any person who isn't here, right now.**

We talk of past aspects and future aspects.

We can be very precise and talk about that aspect of you who was very excited when they were told some good news at 3pm on Wednesday.

This avoids having to squish all these many different people who we really are into a single messy "I."

Instead of thinking/saying, "I am naughty and nice, I am patient and impatient, I am happy and angry, I'm stupid and smart, I'm strong and I'm weak, and none of that makes any sense!"

We say, "I am here. Yesterday around lunch time, my aspect got extremely stressed and did something I wish she had not."

Instead of saying, "Peter is a bully!" we say, "Peter's stressed aspects are bullies. When he's not stressed, his aspects can be really nice."

It takes a little while to get used to referring to one's past aspects and future aspects in that way, but it is well worth it.

For example, a teenage boy was told, "If you leave your shoes there, your aspect tomorrow is going to get all stressed out because he won't find them." For the first time ever, he agreed, picked up his shoes and placed them by his bed – for his morning aspect to find them there.

Relating to aspects, rather than trying to love or forgive "yourself," is much easier and leads to a profound re-unification.

It works with the energy body especially well, as we can direct energy to ourselves in the now, as well as to past aspects and future aspects.

The most important lesson of the Aspects Model is this.

- **Everyone has many aspects, and the more stressed the aspects are, the worse they will behave.**

To understand that someone - your child, your partner, your boss, the checkout assistant, the aggressive driver - is simply stressed makes all the difference.

It makes us instantly more compassionate, more patient, and allows us to respond more accurately and positively.

Instead of getting stressed ourselves and falling to into the same stress pit, we can start to think of new and different ways to deal with any situation.

Sometimes it is just a matter of walking away, but often we can help a stressed person become less stressed - and therefore, a better person.

- **Understanding that everybody can be "good" or "bad" depending where they are on the Energy Chart can also end confusion about "what kind of person you are."**

It can help us break out of labels we have been given, and returns us simply to being a normal human being who reacts predictably when stress gets too high.

Most of all, understanding how energy body stress works in people (and in animals, who also have an energy system) gives us a clear route out of trouble and into much better performance all around.

Feed the energy body with Positives.

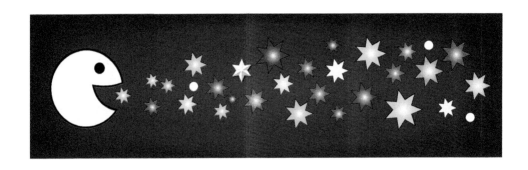

It's as simple as that. And as profound.

And as ... rEvolutionary.

rEvolution

"You find yourself at +10."

Silvia Hartmann

Introduction

- *Based on a transcript of Silvia Hartmann's keynote speech at the 2017 GoE Energy Conference, entitled "The Love Challenge."*

In 2011, I spoke before the GoE Energy Conference and encouraged the participants to come out of the energy closet.

Then, it was thought that if you talked about energy, you would have to be a fool. People were afraid to admit that they were working with energy, reversed to stand up and speak their truth.

I taught the participants to hold out their hands and to say,

"Good morning! My name is ... and I am a Modern Energist!

"It is my job to make people happier."

It helps that the Modern Energy theory I have created is not only reasonable and rational, can be directly observed and measured in a myriad of different ways, but also makes sense to every normal human being on this planet.

Coming out of the energy closet and admitting that we are Modern Energists was the first step into the world on the other side of a major paradigm shift.

- **Understanding the world with 6 senses, rather than five, adds 16.7% additional information.**

The additional 16.7% of information is what connects the dots. These are the missing puzzle pieces that are needed to explain why people do the things they do, why they think and behave the way they do, and what we have to do in order to evolve out of the dark ages of humanity at last.

Modern Energy is an absolute game changer. It is a true paradigm shift; an evolution so radical, we might as well call it a r[E]volution.

In order to understand the origins of the Energy r[E]volution, we have to travel back to 1987, where a past aspect, a young and enthusiastic Silvia Hartmann, was researching animal behaviour, and in particular, the so called "Rage Syndrome."

This is an extreme explosion of rage in managed animals (farm animals, zoo animals, companion animals) which can be dangerous to the keepers, and no way of either understanding or predicting this behaviour had been found.

For the cause of Rage Syndrome, the research team was looking at many factors including diet, husbandry, toxins in the environment, and genetic pre-disposition, but no common causative factor could be found.

The young Hartmann aspect became interested in relational structural patterns, rather than looking at Rage Syndrome in isolation, and found that there was an escalation chain which began with simple "Attention Seeking Behaviour" and led directly to Rage Syndrome as the catastrophic yet entirely predictable outcome.

She theorised that there was something invisible being exchanged between social mammals, and this something invisible had direct, measurable effects on the behaviour of individuals.

She called the invisible something "attention" and created a simple, structural model that worked perfectly to both measure stress states and predict behaviour in social mammals.

The day came, and the aspect had a breakthrough experience and understood that what she had thought of as attention was actually about love.

- **Rage Syndrome in social mammals is caused by an absence of love.**

There is a very real energy exchange going on between social mammals, and when this energy exchange is disturbed or disrupted, terrible things happen.

Terrible, terrible things.

There was a study about orphans at the beginning of the 20th Century, where nurses were allowed to feed and change orphaned babies, but they were not allowed to interact with them beyond that. No eye contact, the nurses wore gloves and did not speak.

At first, the babies, although well fed and clean, started to cry hysterically, incessantly. What happened next was that the babies stopped crying. Then they stopped eating, and then they started dying.

At which point the nurses, even back then, refused to take further part and so the experiment was never completed.

- **This energy exchange between social mammals is a structural occurrence and not limited to people. These energy exchanges happen between horses, monkeys, dolphins, cats, dogs, rats, elephants, meerkats and lions.**

- **All the social mammals have these energy exchanges happening between them, and these energy exchanges are absolutely crucial to their intelligence, their social functioning, their physical health, their powers of recovery, to their emotional health, to their behaviour, how they react in any given environment and how they behave with each other.**

In a flash, my aspect saw the effects of lack of love on social mammals.

Yes, and there is the story of how my 1993 aspect ran into the room with the animal behaviour library, which contained everything that had ever been published in the English language on animal behaviour, every book, every paper, every article, every scientific study.

She took one book after the other from the shelf and searched for this, but the word LOVE wasn't in any of them.

Not one occurrence, not in any of them.

There was a mountain of scientific books at the aspect's feet, and the word LOVE was not in any of them.

In that moment, I understood why the world of humans was in such a mess.

The most important factor of them all was missing from all the scientific equations constructed in the "age of reason."

I also understood there was nothing more important in the world than to correct this horrific oversight that had made science as it stands entirely illogical.

That is where I come from – to bring LOVE into science, to create a new science that includes love.

All the various techniques I have tested and researched over the decades have never been only about tapping, or EMO, or any of that.

- **The core drive is to re-combine LOVE and LOGIC.**

It is of the essence to bring that missing 16.7% of information about energy, about love, into science because without it, you cannot understand people.

The energy body is real and it creates all our emotions, and you cannot make sense of people at all without factoring in emotions.

Further, people themselves cannot make sense of the Universe at large without factoring in the additional information set provided by their own emotions.

Yes, and so I brought down this whole story to emotions being feedback devices from the real, true, living energy body.

- **When the energy body is happy, we experience happy emotions.**
- **When the energy body is unhappy or in pain, we experience negative emotions.**

From EMO we know that the exact place where we feel our emotional pain is the exact place where the disturbance in the energy body is located.

"Where do you feel this heartbreak in your body? Show me with your hands!"

We don't have to guess, we don't have to intuit, people can show us where it hurts, and that's the place that needs healing.

We can put our healing hands of energy over that place and find out what happens next …

When we take the energy body seriously, all of a sudden emotions make sense. They become structural, systemic, and predictable.

We have the beginnings of a rational, logical new science of energy – The Third Field.

Going back to the original desire to bring love back into science, of course it was all about love. That was the word the aspects used. But then the aspects changed their terminology to be less offensive – instead of love, we talk about energy.

The State Of Play

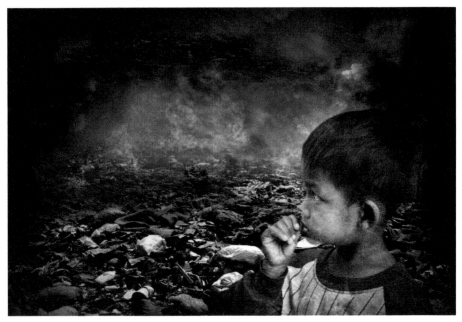

The world of men is a mess – and it's not getting any better.

Wherever you look, there is a nightmare unfolding that destroys human lives in any way you might want to conceive of it.

The problems are so many, so grandiose, so intense, they are frightening and overwhelming.

In the picture above, we see a little child looking at a burning heap of garbage.

In the so-called civilised world, we live in the illusion that things are getting better. We live in our clean cities with street lights and spend our time sending each other motivational pictures on social media. Every year, a slew of new gadgets come out and we can celebrate that – it's progress.

Things are getting better …

No, they are not getting better - and there is one particular topic that breaks into that illusion of the world of people.

The Trillion Dollar Stress Pandemic

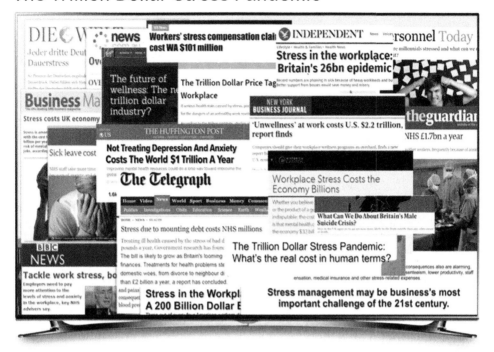

The so-called civilised world is breaking down under the chronic stress of its inhabitants.

For all the yoga, consumption of organic foods, recycling and wearing exercise watches that tell us how many steps we've walked today, stress is rising and rising – and so is the cost of stress.

Here is something that cannot be ignored any longer, because it is starting to hit the illusion where it hurts – in the accumulation of profits.

To be sure, the Trillion Dollar Stress Pandemic isn't nearly as expensive as all the money spent on the tools and toys of war. It is a drop in the ocean compared to the complete insanity of that.

The problem is however that the stress problem is personal. People have real experience of stress, what it does to their lives. Stress is not as easily ignored as wars fought far away in foreign countries, or little foreign children looking at the destruction of their environments.

Stress is a real problem and there is no solution to be found for this in the illusionary non-reality of the world of people that tries to pretend there's no such thing as ENERGY.

A 2023 Comment: I was deeply concerned about the effects of stress in 2014 as I noted how much more stressed and insane public discourse was starting to become.

People becoming more chaotic, more volatile, more extreme in their thinking and behaviours and all manner of mental disturbances being on the rise showed clearly that we were living in a trillion dollar stress pandemic.

Just when you thought it couldn't get any worse, it got a lot worse. Everyone's life was destroyed during the global panic pandemic 2020 to 2022, and now we are beyond a stress catastrophe.

Still, nobody is actively addressing this in any meaningful way.

The Modern Energy rEvolution is needed more now than ever before.

Please pass on the essential message that we have living energy bodies which are real, and which produce symptoms, cries of pain, which cannot be controlled with pills, potions, injections or putting a chip in the brain.

This is important.

There is nothing any one of us can do about so many things that threaten our health and our sanity.

But we can do something about the state of our own energy bodies.

In order to do that, we must understand that energy bodies are real.

The Mysterious Energy Body

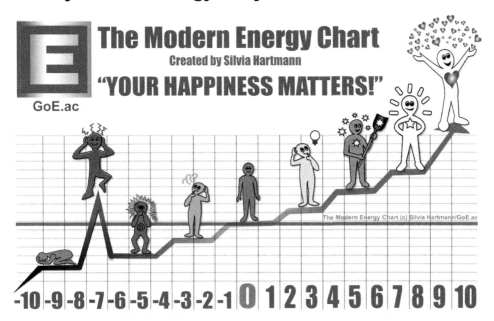

As Modern Energists, we have an entire set of new theories, methodologies and techniques to address stress in a whole new way.

This is a proven and effective way; we've been doing this for 25 years now and we know that it works.

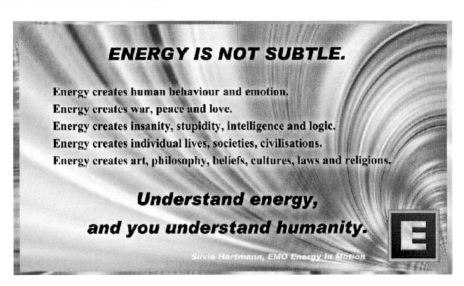

Energy Is Not Subtle!

It all starts with the idea, "YES! You really have an energy body!"

Followed by,

"And NO, it's not that wibbly wobbly thing from the old New Age, that is so abstract that you have to meditate to see auras and lick flowers.

"NO! It's not one of those weird things with a billion points, thin needly little lines, or chakras stacked up like dinner plates!

"NO! I am not talking about some sort of subtle energy body!

"I'm talking about the energy body that makes a man punch his wife in the face and knock her teeth out.

"I'm talking about the sort of energy body that makes a person jump off a motorway bridge, because they can't stand the pain of living any longer, and cause an accident that kills six hundred people, including a school bus full of kids.

"I am talking about the energy body that makes people want to go to war.

"I am talking about the energy body that when it lights up properly creates the sort of person that starts a religion which lasts for a thousand years and involves billions!

"That's the sort of energy body I'm talking about!"

People hear this and are astonished.

They say, "What, you mean a real energy body?"

I say, "Yes. **A real energy body**. With an energy head, and energy organs, energy veins and arteries, energy digestion system and healing hands of energy!

"That real energy body expresses itself in emotions, and depending on how well the energy body functions, how high or low your energy body states are, is not only how you feel, and how you act, but also what structural grammar you are using in your language; what beliefs you hold, and those are different between the different energy body states, and your entire physical body chemistry changes as well."

The Modern Energy Chart gives us an overview of the different energy body states we can inhabit, from -10 to +10.

The fact is that every normal human being will have been in all of these states at some point in their lives, no matter how briefly.

The Modern Energy Chart doesn't describe 9 different people – it only shows ONE, and this one person goes up and down like a yo-yo all the time, every day, all through their lives.

We have had aspects that were on top of the world; we have had aspects who succeeded. We have also had aspects who were so broken down, they lay down on the floor and cried.

We have had aspects who were truly terrified; aspects who questioned themselves.

We have been bored and lifeless, uninspired and grey.

We have had aspects who had good ideas, and we have had aspects who went out to work on a project, full of excitement and energy.

We have had aspects who were walking on water because they were in love, and aspects who couldn't breathe from the pain of a broken heart.

This is good and right.

I do not believe that we're supposed to be floating around locked into a constant state of +10 all the time. Human experience covers the range and makes us real, makes us wise. The most fertile landscapes exist where the weather changes, where there is sunshine and rain, thunderstorms and blue skies – all of it.

So essentially, we want to embrace the entire range of human experiences, but there is a huge problem.

- **The problem is that we do not seem to be having nearly enough good experiences on the positive side of the Energy Chart.**

This is curious, as every human being lives and strives all the time for better experiences, better emotions.

What has happened to people?

Where are the good experiences, the high energy experiences we could and should be having every day of our lives?

Where did the good emotions go???

It is a question that has troubled me deeply for quite some time now.

The Evil Scissors

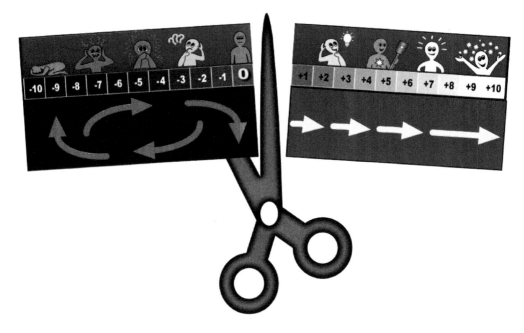

I said in conversation not long ago that it seemed to me that at some point, someone came along with a great big pair of evil scissors, cut that scale in half - and then threw the good half away!

All we're left with is that crazy negative side.

The good side, the positive side, is … absent???

How can that be true?

It seems truly crazy, but it is.

For example, here is a pain assessment tool from medical practice.

The Pain Assessment Tool

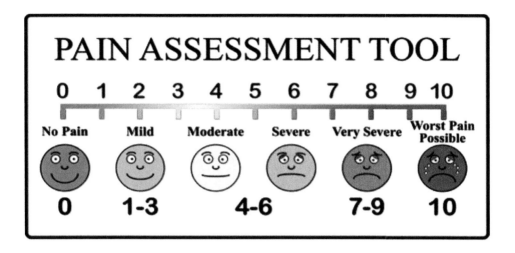

It goes from 10, what we would call -10, and ends at ZERO – **no pain**.

This scale is missing the positive side altogether.

Surely, beyond simply feeling no pain, feeling nothing, there is more to be had?

Shouldn't there be a state where the body feels good, then great, then spectacular – and THAT is the truly healed state?

Are the goal posts for physical medicine set way too low?

Are people sent home way too early in medical treatments, halfway through, without a real healing ever having been reached ..?

The SUD Scale

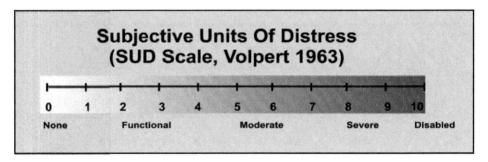

And then we have the Subjective Units of Distress scale (SUD Scale), an old psychology instrument clearly copied straight across from the medical pain scale.

Again, we are only measuring pain, and we're not measuring pleasure here.

Indeed, exactly as with the medical pain chart, the positive side of this scale is simply absent.

It isn't there. It doesn't exist at all.

This is a conceptual nightmare.

Medicine might get away with it, but to try and understand people this is blatantly a pack of cards with all the trumps removed.

When I started to work with people, I asked them a question nobody else had asked. I would ask a sex abuse victim, "So what was good about it?" They would be astonished and taken aback, but I would ask again, "What was good about it?"

And the person might say, "Well, there was the ice cream and feeling special. And most of all, knowing more than all the other children. They knew nothing, but I knew everything."

Now, we have a bigger picture. Now, we know more than we did before that question was asked. We have more information than we did when we only asked about the pain.

This was when I found the Guiding Stars, the high positive experiences that cause a person to repeat the same behaviours over and over again.

The classic example is that of a boy who sees his mother's high heeled shoe, has his first sexual experience and now he's a shoe collector, age 43, with 123,000 pairs of high heeled shoes. He has no wife, no love life, no life at all, no friends, but he has shoes – and it comes straight from that one highly positive experience. Guiding Stars create loops from which a person cannot escape unless their energy system is addressed.

Unless you understand both trauma and Guiding Star, you can never understand a person as there is an interplay between positive and negative experiences.

And once you start investigating people's Guiding Stars, we're in a whole new world of human experiences, where there is so much more to be learned, to be discovered – including the real Star Events.

The Yerkes Dobson Law Of Arousal

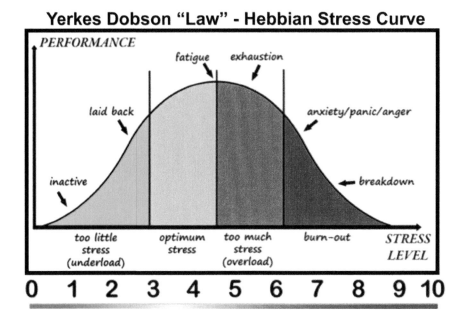

Yerkes Dobson "Law" - Hebbian Stress Curve

Here is a third example of that missing positive wing which exists in the Energy Chart.

When I was writing the Modern Stress Management materials, I decided to have a look what the current standard of Stress Research might be at, and I found "The Yerkes Dobson LAW of Arousal."

Here, we have two American scientists in 1908 (yes, 1908!) and their rats.

These guys had a sleeping rat in a cage, and they would electro-shock it and open a door to a maze, and then measure how long it took for the rat to get to the end of the maze.

If they didn't shock the rat enough, the rat would go back to sleep.

If they shocked the rat too much, it would freak out completely and throw itself around like a lunatic, and that would be our -7, where the Rage Syndrome was found.

If they shocked the rats just enough, the rat would wake up in a panic and try to run away as fast as it could in sheer terror.

From this our friends Yerkes and Dobson created THE LAW OF AROUSAL 1908. On this "scientific" basis, people have been stressing their workers, their soldiers, their school children and presumably their scientists, to drive them into what they called optimal stress – which is actually our -4 and -5 stress, and what we call severe and debilitating chronic stress.

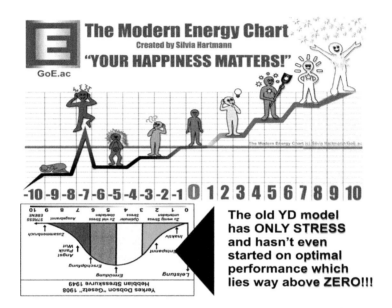

What Yerkes and Dobson failed to do was to let the rats have a good night's sleep, and let them wake up naturally. To give them a good breakfast – and then put a female rat at the end of that maze. They never did that experiment, but I guarantee that those happy rats would have produced better results in terms of learning the maze, the speed and elegance of their movements and how fast they would get there, reliably, every single time.

There is a pattern here that is is deeply disturbing.

The Wall At ZERO

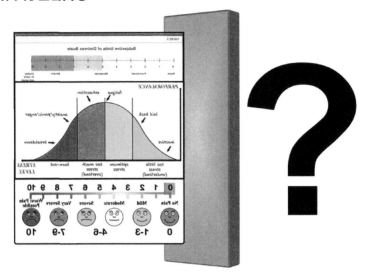

The pattern that is being revealed here is that there is a gigantic barrier at ZERO. This barrier keeps people trapped on the wrong side of the Energy Chart.

This is **a conceptual prison** - the good stuff isn't there, doesn't even exist conceptually.

A most current example of this is research into chronic pain being conducted right now at a prestigious university in the UK.

The researchers have found that the "mood" of the patient influences the brain activity relating to the experience of chronic pain.

For their research, they have subjects focus on something that makes them sad or angry (the negative side) and compare this with clients who are relaxed or resting (the Zero state).

They find that the Zero state subjects experience less pain and the brain scans show a difference in brain activity.

What they are NOT researching however, is what would happen if a third group was tested, who were happy – energy high, as we would say.

The "mood" changes the experience of chronic pain in the brain.		You didn't even think to try ...
Negative Mood Anger, Sadness	Neutral Mood Feeling nothing	Positive Mood? Happiness, Laughter, LOVE?

More Pain	**Less Pain**	**??????????**

In not even considering that 3rd option from the other side of the great wall of Zero, the chronic pain researchers are missing out on the most important information, the most relevant data; in fact they are failing to find the exact mechanism that could potentially lead to a breakthrough in chronic pain management, the greater questions on how the brain works, and a Nobel prize at the end.

We have that same conceptual problem yet again that you will find absolutely everywhere, once you start to notice this.

- **Nobody is looking beyond ZERO, nobody is researching beyond ZERO, and this has some truly nasty repercussions for humanity at large.**

War, Peace, ...???

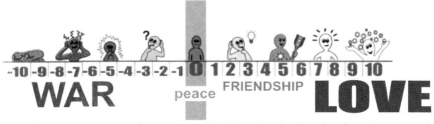

War and peace are a perfect example. War is obviously the -7 state when entire groups or whole civilisations completely lose the plot and starting to mindlessly and senselessly attack each other. But what is peace? Peace is simply the absence of war - a true ZERO state where nothing is gained, nothing is achieved, nothing is CREATED, where there is no evolution. This is extremely unattractive to modern human beings as a goal in and of itself, but it gets even worse.

- **The balance point between war and peace is at -4.**

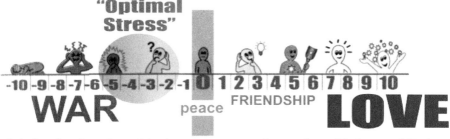

Isn't it fascinating that -4 is the exact same place where Yerkes and Dobson had their stressed rats trying to escape the terror, and on the Modern Energy Chart, the place where self doubt turns into fear and paranoia. It's little wonder that we have so much war, are always on the brink of war, and are constantly cycling round and round in the "war & peace" version of the fish tank of insanity, with no way out in sight!

A true balance needs that other side of the chart being present, but of course, it isn't there.

Peace is the ZERO point of nothing. If you want to end war, you don't need peace as a goal. You need a much higher goal. You need LOVE as the goal at +10. When you fall short of that, at least we might be on the right side of the chart and can come up with some creative, practical solutions to the problems that caused the wars in the first place.

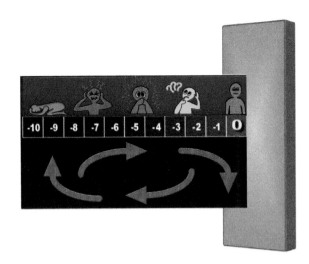

The direct result of the conceptual absence of the good side of the Energy Chart causes this crazy wall at ZERO.

Trapped on the negative side, everyone is circling round and round and round, repeating the old over and over and over again with no way out, no progress in sight.

It's worse than no progress as well.

The longer it goes on, the more destructive the absence of the positive side becomes on those poor energy bodies, trapped on the wrong side behind the ZERO barrier, and the crazier human beings must become.

Here is an amazing example of how this plays out in practice.

The Cult Of Trauma

A great example on how this works with real people is that of a cult who took the (wrongful, destructive, erroneous) idea that we are basically perfect but then were messed up by trauma entirely seriously and ran with it.

The idea is that if we remove all the trauma, we become "clear" - perfect beings in mind, body and spirit.

So they would find people who were highly stressed, around -5 or -6, and gave them some focused attention and hope. In other words, they would raise people's energy bodies up the energy chart with social energy and direct them towards a future where things might be better.

This would produce "gains" – the person would move up on the energy chart and start to feel a little bit better.

That proves the theory, right?

So all we have to do now is go on clearing trauma, and at the end, when there is no trauma left, we will have superhuman abilities, we'll never get sick ever again, and become the masters of the Universe.

So the members of the trauma cult went at it and cleared their traumas – only, they didn't really clear anything because all they were looking for was that at the end of the session, they should feel nothing at all. ZERO emotions.

ZERO for the energy body is exactly that – nothing. In order to heal or evolve the energy body, you need high positive outcomes, but in that crazy world where everything stops at ZERO, that idea doesn't even exist.

More and more traumas were being taken to ZERO.

The gains started to flatten out, until there were no more gains at all.

At which point someone might have had the bright idea to ask, "Wait a minute – is there something else beyond clearing trauma to ZERO? Something other than trauma? Something beyond ZERO?"

Nobody did.

So they decided there had to have been more trauma, only perhaps it wasn't the trauma we remembered, but instead, trauma we didn't remember.

That opened up a whole new realm of trauma clearance, as people started to hallucinate problems they never had, "false memory syndrome" came into being and more and more trauma appeared like the shards of the sorcerer's apprentices broom - but the gains didn't materialise.

Still, nobody questioned the central idea that by clearing trauma we become perfect. This was still the gospel, so it was just that the real trauma had not yet been found …

Ah! Perhaps it is pre-natal trauma …

Same story.

Ah! Perhaps it is past life trauma …

Now things are starting to get crazy. Instead of further gains, people are starting to get strange new symptoms, getting ever more stressed, getting ill, acting strangely, definitely thinking very strange thoughts …

Where is the trauma???

Ah! Brilliant idea! It's alternate life trauma! And this could also include alternate past lives as well as alternate future lives … and now it's endless …

Trapped behind that ZERO barrier, with no way out, with nobody saying, "For the love of God, stop it with the trauma!" things were only going to get crazier and crazier.

Let me say this clearly and succinctly.

- **Trauma is not what shapes our lives.**

It is but a minute component; but by giving it all that focused attention, and blaming everything on trauma we have created an entirely imaginary demon to battle in a hideous labyrinth of trauma and more trauma from which there is literally no escape – ever.

Every time we talk about trauma, think about trauma, connect with trauma, we're bringing our energy bodies down and causing additional stress to an already highly unstable system that nobody even knows exists!

To start to look beyond trauma is what is desperately needed today to save us all from the crazy, dangerous stress overload we find ourselves in.

The Fish Tank Of Insanity

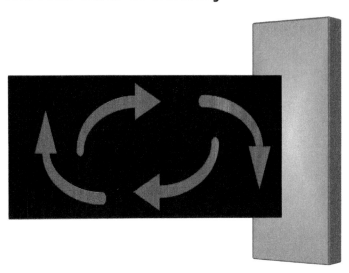

Running up against the conceptual ZERO barrier and cycling round and round between nothing and trauma, nothing and war, between nothing and stress, between nothing and pain, has created what I call **the fish tank of insanity**.

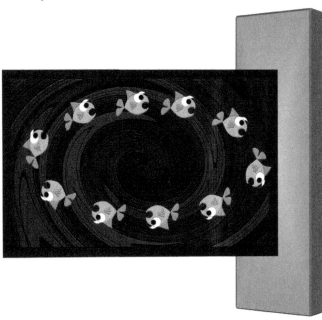

What is so crazy about this fish tank of insanity is that it is an **entirely conceptual prison** – it doesn't exist outside the minds of human beings who have lost the plot and the entire positive side of the Modern Energy Chart.

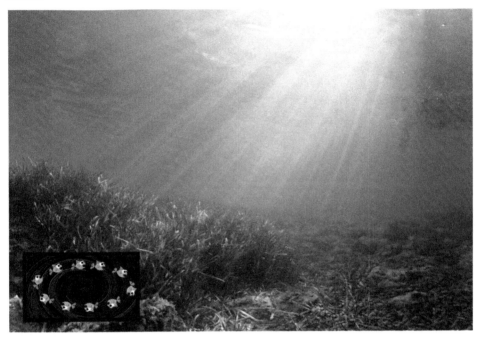

There is nothing truthful or logical about the fish tank of insanity.

The real truth is that people experience positive emotions as well and all the time.

The world doesn't stop at ZERO – the really real word, that would be.

The real world includes highs and lows and everything in between.

The real world, and especially the Oceans of Energy, is endlessly abundant.

- **We start waking up to the real world, and our place within it, on the other side of grand barrier at ZERO.**

Free The Fish!

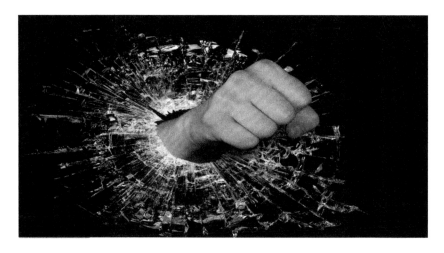

As a Modern Energist, I hold it to be my purpose and mission to punch through that ZERO barrier so that …

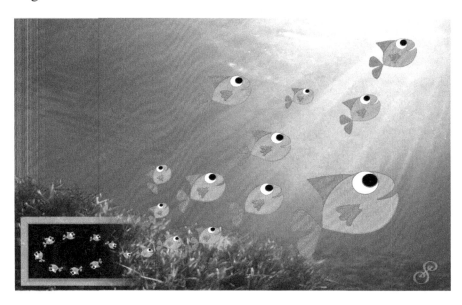

The fish can swim free!
Yes, that's the rEvolution!

Choose Your Plane ...

Now I would personally like to free humanity from the crazy stress riddled fish tank of insanity all at once, but for now, I would be happy if individuals understood that there is a choice to be made, and then go ahead and make that choice.

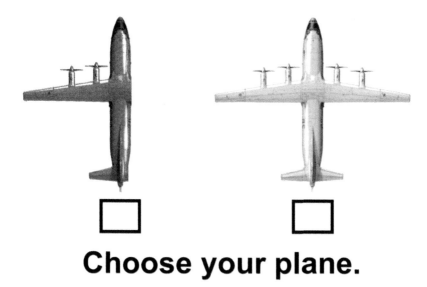

Choose your plane.

At the moment, people don't realise that there is this whole other world out there that holds the answers not only to almost all of their problems, but also to almost all of their life long questions.

At the moment, almost every psychology based counselling session anywhere delves only into trauma and negative emotions of the past.

At the moment, every single stress program in the whole world drives people deeper into stress, by wrongfully placing "peak performance" at -4 instead of where it belongs, at +10.

At the moment, the people of the world are praying for peace to try and end the endless wars, when they should be praying for LOVE instead. Even when someone dies, people are saying, "Rest in peace," when they should be saying, "Soar in joy!" instead.

At the moment, people are endlessly disempowered by the conceptual absence of the positive wing of the Energy Chart, having lost access to the source of their own personal power.

At the moment, trauma and victimhood are wrongfully elevated to high status, and when people talk about "lived experience," all they talk about is trauma.

At the moment, people are endlessly separated from each other because you need to be energy high to make true connections between one another.

- **Trapped on the wrong side of the Energy Chart, people are alone.**

This is perhaps the greatest catastrophe for humanity of them all.

Disconnection

The more stressed and energy poor the energy body becomes, the more weak and fragile it becomes in turn. Below Zero, the energy body has collapsed to the point that we no longer energetically connect with our environments, and that includes all of creation, the Oceans of Energy, and most of all, each other.

⭐ **Below Zero, we are structurally disconnected from one another.**

The more stressed they are, the more disconnected individuals become from one another.

This precludes people from working together to find solutions for our global problems; it also precludes understanding each other, having sympathy for each other, and it leads to people feeling powerless, unloved and alone.

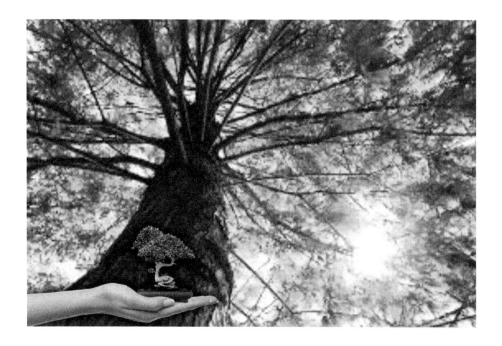

I have likened what happens to the human energy body under chronic stress to what happens when you put a tree into a very small pot and cut off its roots and branches.

Not only does this lead to a severe shrinking of the entire energy system, and what we end up with is nothing at all like the natural order of things.

Where there could have been a mighty tree, we have an impoverished version that isn't even a shadow of what it should have been. What also happens is that every little bonsai tree is all alone in its little pot. In the real world, where the trees go large and to the light, their leaves touch each other, their roots form connections and the trees are not alone.

We often talk about potential and wonder how far we humans can truly go.

We wonder how to activate and actualise our true potential.

Expanding our energy systems, setting our energy bodies free to grow and expand with proper energy nutrition is definitely a step in the right direction.

Finding Yourself

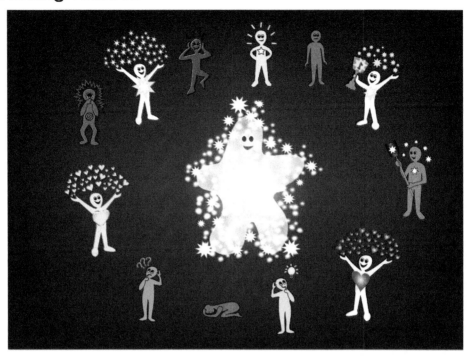

⭐ **You find out who you really are at +10, and <u>only at +10</u>.**

Anything else is an impoverished version of you, a stressed version.

Your true self as well as your true potential becomes revealed when the energy system reaches its true Even Flow – and that's not sitting in the lotus position, gazing at your own navel and dreaming of better days.

At +10, when our energy body works exactly the way it was designed to work in the first place, we find ourselves.

We find the truth about human beings, we become truly loving – and finally also, truly logical.

Love at ZERO is ZERO love!

And …

Logic at ZERO is ZERO logic!

At +10, love & logic are one and the same.

The Lily Story

Someone once confronted me and told me that I was completely deluded to think that "we are who we really are at +10 and nowhere else." That it was just a stupid idea and I was wrong, that the only way to the truth was through suffering, that you could only find out who you really are at -10, not +10. And that the real truth about people was that they were cruel and sin filled, worse than animals, that they were monsters.

I have to admit, I got angry and I said, quite powerfully, "Right. Imagine yourself in an ancient forest, with shafts of golden sunlight streaming through the cathedral trees.

"And there is a gorgeous stand of forest lilies, in their full expression of what lily plants can be - beautiful flowers, glossy leaves, strong roots.

"Then you jump on them, and you kick them, and you trample them more and more and stomp them into the dirt until there's nothing left but a disgusting mess - and you are standing there and seriously telling me that that disgusting mess is the true nature of the lilies?

"Don't you dare!"

The person in question stared at me for a good long time, eyes wide open, Adams apple going up and down quite remarkably, and then said weakly, "Oh ... " followed by, "So that's what you mean ..."

Damn right that's what I mean.

A person doesn't know who they are until and unless they experienced their +10 aspects. Everything else is a stressed, distorted, disturbed version of their own true self. That's the truth.

As modern energists, we know this. We've had our own +10s and we know what that does to you, how that makes you feel, how that makes you *be* and how that makes you be-have.

The +10 is quite real. There is a +10 for every aspect, and these +10s evolve as we evolve, with experience and practice.

We need to want them, we need to seek them, we need to embrace them - and we need to learn to re-reverse that enormous global reversal of our stress-riddled societies and "look for the good."

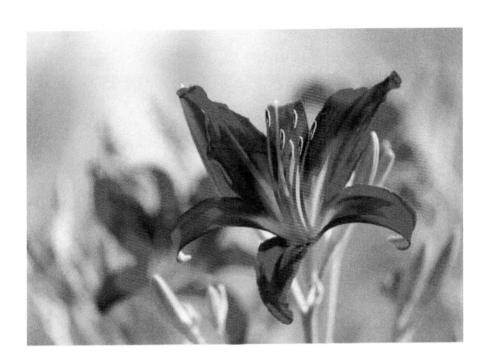

You start seeking the good, and it will find you.

You start seeking the magic, and it will find you.

You start seeking the truth - and it *will* find you.

The Undiscovered Country Of Love

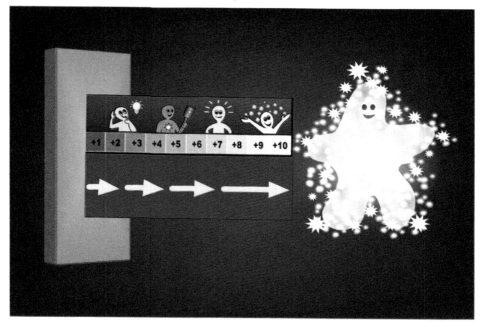

The most important message of Modern Energy is this.

To answer our most urgent questions, to solve our most urgent problems, but at the end of the day, to get out of that state of endless chronic stress, fire fighting, endless struggle and quite literally, the rat race in which humanity has been caught for far too long, **we need to explore the positive wing of the Energy Chart.**

> ✯ **Everything that is good, right, holy, healing, logical, truthful, powerful and enlightening lies on the other side of the great ZERO barrier.**

We need to start exploring what is going on in this totally undiscovered country of POSITIVE energy states with all urgency and with all speed.

As anything to do with energy is currently scientific heresy in the so called "age of reason," we can't sit back and wait for the great minds in their ivory towers who are supposed to do all the thinking on behalf of the rest of us to finally see the light.

Each one of us – you, me, him and her over there as well – need to start realising that our energy bodies are real, that they have been trying to communicate with us all our lives, and above all else, we have to start realising that "our happiness MATTERS."

Contrary to current opinion, it is not our suffering that will lead us towards our own personal happiness, however each one of us wants to define that at the moment.

Suffering begets more suffering, and so does dwelling on the suffering.

The only way forward is to move towards happiness – towards more energy, towards more power, towards more LOVE.

Everything Changes ...

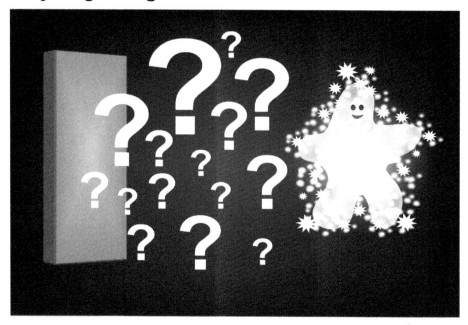

The Power of the Positives has been ignored for far too long.

Understanding that literally **everything** changes when people become not emotionally balanced, but simply happier, is of the essence.

⭐ **When our energy body states change, our entire body chemistry changes.**

An aspect at -8 has a totally different body chemistry than an aspect of the exact same person who is at +8.

As a result, these different aspects (of the same person!) will react completely differently to all manner of physical substances.

Indeed, we would need to re-run every single medical experiment related to the effects of drugs on human beings because it was never factored in what energy body state the test subjects were in.

Give a -8 person an aspirin, and their reaction will be completely different from those of a +8 person. The very physical change in body chemistry that is the direct result of an energy body state change also gives us a myriad of new and promising research directions.

What does a +8 person have in their blood that a -8 person does not? And vice versa? There is so much that we must learn with great urgency to find better ways of treating not just the energy body, but also the physical body, as a direct result of factoring in energy at last.

In the meantime, each one of us has their own living energy body, and their own energy body needs.

Every one of us can do simple things right now to start a true Renaissance of their energy body, and reap multiple benefits from doing so.

Each one of us can undertake their own journey of discovery, their own journey into the amazing land on the other side of that ZERO barrier, to find out new things about what we can do when we become more energy rich in our daily lives.

The Healing Energy Remedies

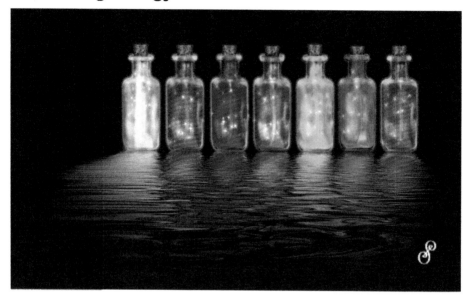

An entire lifetime of neglecting and not understanding the needs of the energy body has left us with all sorts of problems and in that constant state of fire fighting, circling around in our fish tank of insanity on the wrong side of ZERO.

> ⭐ **<u>Everyone</u> needs urgent energy remedies and essential energy nutrition for their energy body, <u>right now</u>.**

It is literally of the essence that we start to ask ourselves every day, "What I do I need? What do I want?" and finally listen and pay attention to the needs of our energy bodies.

We need to understand that we can't fix our energy bodies with material stuff, with objects, with chemicals, with substances.

The things we need and which are described in words such as JOY, PASSION, RESPECT, POWER, LOVE, EXCITEMENT, ADVENTURE, HAPPINESS are all **ENERGY**.

> ⭐ **The vitamins the energy body needs are what we call The Positives.**

We can energy tap these, EMO these or simply turn our hearts and minds towards the Positives to raise energy and do something good for our starving energy bodies.

"What do I need? What would help me solve this problem? If only I had more (COURAGE, CONFIDENCE, STRENGTH, HELP, SUPPORT, I need a MIRACLE!) …"

We need to re-train ourselves to search for the Positives we need to make our energy bodies stronger, instead of reflexively flipping back into the past and going on some crazy journey through the trauma nightmare labyrinth that gets us nowhere.

We need to learn to be far more flexible in our approaches and ask often, pay attention all the time, and then actually use the extraordinary powers of positive energy to heal, rejuvenate and revitalise our energy bodies.

Energy Intelligence

Our living energy bodies react IMMEDIATELY when we "think about something."

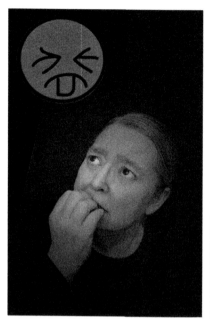 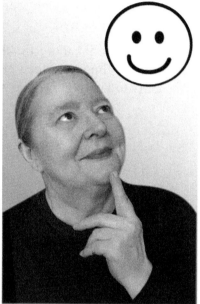

- When we think about something good, we go up on the Energy Chart.
- When we think about something bad, we go down.

It's instant, and reliable.

This being so, we want to engage this Super Power of our conscious minds in the right way to keep our dear living energy bodies from getting too stressed.

Constantly watching bad news, getting into fights with others, worrying about major ongoings that are completely outside our power to do anything about them, dwelling on trauma and insults is really, really bad for the energy body, especially long term.

I am not saying that we shouldn't be thinking about our problems; but what I am saying is that thinking about problems while we are in low energy states is worse than just being a complete waste of time.

Literally, nothing good can come of it. The lower our energy states are, the more idiotic our attempts at fixing our problems become, and the less likely they are to do anything good for anyone at all.

Energy intelligence begins when we become consciously aware how our own thoughts, actions and reactions in daily life determine the fate of our own living energy bodies.

We need to move from having ignored our energy bodies to putting them first instead. Yes, they really are that important. Some might think if you are caught in a burning building, the last thing you want to be doing is to think of something positive to raise your energy – but even there, stumbling around blindly as a stress crazy fool is not going to save your life or keep you safe.

You have a better chance with an energy body in a higher state – and that is energy intelligence at work.

Learn To Raise Your Energy

⭐ **A huge part of the Energy rEvolution is to stop putting up with low energy states all the time.**

We must stop believing it is good to be stressed, that it is normal to worry and feel miserable, that it is right to be scared all the time, or that we have to suffer for whatever crazy reasons because it is good to be suffering.

All of that is of the old; it is understandable and a direct result of being trapped in those negative energy states, the lore of the fish tank of insanity, but it has to stop now.

We have to start picking up our power to take energy from the endlessly abundant, overflowing Oceans of Energy and use this to make ourselves happier.

We have to counteract the entrainments and habits of a lifetime and start to ask ourselves, "What do I need to be happier? Stronger? More playful? More joyful? How can I make my life more effortless, more beautiful, more exciting? What do I need right now to cheer up?"

When we have the answer, we need to not just nod and say, "Oh that makes sense ..."

We actually have to do something about it!

A Practical Application: Raising Energy With Love

Here is a simple Modern Energy Exercise that anyone can do to raise energy noticeably.

Try it out for yourself, right now.

Step 1: Take an energy reading: Where are you on the Modern Energy Chart, right now?

Slide your finger over the SUE Scale and find your number.

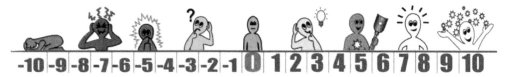

Step 2: Assume the Heart Position and take three deep breaths, in and out.

The Heart Position

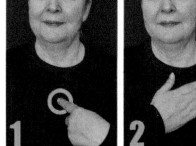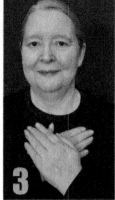

Point to the place where you would point and say, "This is me!" That is the centre of your heart of energy.

- Place the centre of the palm of your leading hand over that spot.
- Put your other hand on top.
- Take three deep breaths, in and out.

Now think of someone or something you love as you continue to breathe deeply for one minute.

Step 3: Take a new energy reading.

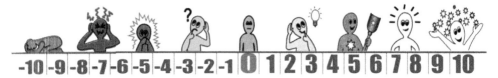

Congratulations! You have raised energy by using the power of love.

START with the HEART!

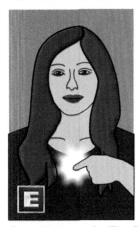
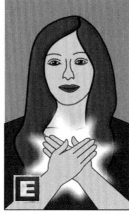

Brought to you by The Guild of Energists GoE.ac
"We LOVE Energy!"

- Nervous?
- Anxious?
- Stressed out?
- Freaked out?
- Upset?
- Distraught?
- Depressed?

START with the HEART!

Point to yourself, "This is me!"
- Place your leading hand's palm over that spot.
- Now place your other hand on top.
- Focus on the sensations of your hands on your chest.
- Breathe in deeply.
- Breathe out slowly.   *Share*
- This helps you centre.

The Heart of Energy is the power source at the centre of your energy system.

Look after your heart and remember:

START with the HEART.

Simply placing your own healing hands on your own heart of energy and thinking about something or someone you love will raise your energy.

Modern Energy Techniques are all designed to help us revitalise our energy bodies and empower us in the real sense of the word.

Modern Energy Tapping is a quick and easy way to get started on providing our energy bodies with the energy nutrition they need to get stronger and grow up at last.

Modern Stress Management helps us become far more energy aware and gives us new tools and techniques to interact differently with one another, raise each others energy, and create much more harmonious couple bubbles, family bubbles and group bubbles.

EMO Energy In Motion is the engine behind all of Modern Energy. EMO is natural and much faster as we learn to suck in powerful nature energies that are all around us, all the time – accessing the Oceans of Energy in which we live with volition.

Hands of Power finally brings hands on energy healing into the 21st Century once we realise that the hands of our energy body (the energy hands!) are what touches the energy body of another person, and creates changes at that level. This stops all the healing related confusions of the ages and makes direct energy healing safe, logical and effective. And, as this is Modern Energy, instead of only healing, we can do just so much more with our Hands of Power.

SuperMind finally brings our own Energy Minds into play and gives us the ability to transfer our consciousness to an energy rich environment which affects the energy body directly and deals with disturbances in the energy body's neurology as well as providing essential energy nutrition any time this is needed.

Star Matrix is the latest and simplest path yet to be discovered out of that fish tank of insanity - Star Matrix ends the nightmare of trauma, creates a brand new shiny self concept and empowers people in the most extraordinary way, by focusing their attention on their own Star Memories, the best memories, the Treasures & Riches, of their own lives.

There is **Modern Energy Art** to evoke powerful Positives that become real objects, real energy generators that can help us and everyone around us feel better and become stronger.

⭐ **There are a myriad of ways we can gain better energy states.**

The Modern Energy Chart in and of itself gives us many opportunities to use our own experience and intelligence to change the way we react to other people and gain more energy through positive, beneficial interactions which is so essential for a social species like ourselves.

> **Learning to direct attention towards uplifting and life giving energy exchanges in the real world is at the end of the day what drawing on the Powers of The Positives is all about.**

> **Once you understand just how much "your happiness MATTERS," we are a totally different position to take our lives in the right direction – towards true evolution, to become the best person we can be.**

The Power of The Positives

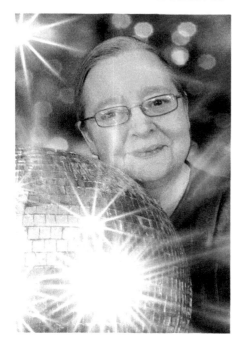

What we call a POSITIVE in Modern Energy is anything that raises <u>YOUR</u> energy.

There are things you, personally, can think about and when you do, you can immediately notice that you start to "feel better."

- **Those things that make YOU feel better are your personal Positives.**

It doesn't matter if other people say something is a Positive for them, or if everyone else says something is positive – in Modern Energy, all your Positives are only Positives if they have a positive effect on YOUR energy body.

Getting to know your own Positives is the first step on a wonderful journey which will grow your ability to improve your energy states, and therefore, your life.

Many people (but of course, not all people!) experience NATURE as a powerful personal Positive.

When they are stressed, they can think about NATURE in general, or even better, personal favourites such as oceans, mountains, animals, flowers and so on, and right away they can notice that they are starting to feel better.

This is taking control of your thoughts and your states of being in a new way.

By practising with your Positives, you will also learn at the same time what you probably shouldn't be thinking, because it's making you feel worse.

- **Our precious, living energy bodies need our attention.**

We cannot go on putting them through hell all the time by uncontrolled, stressed-out thinking which sets up a vicious circle of distress in the energy body, causing even more out of control stressed thinking, which makes the energy body even worse!

Almost the entire population of Planet Earth is doing exactly that right now, and it has got to stop, because the human cost is absolutely incalculable – and this is entirely unnecessary suffering!

The Positives, YOUR Positives, are the way out of these awful stress loops that lead to ill health, insanity, broken relationships, bad luck, bad decisions, bad behaviour, mistakes, accidents and so much more.

- **The Positives are the way out of stress, and towards your personal happiness.**

The Battle For The Positives

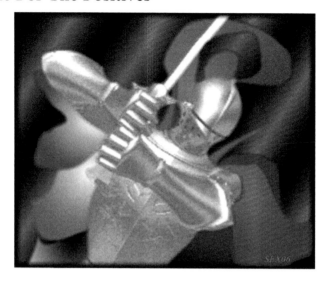

When you start talking about Positive Energy, many people will immediately roll their eyes and declare that you must be incredibly stupid, naïve, deluded, weak willed and utterly unscientific, utterly non-realistic.

That you must be some kind of unicorn loving snowflake holistic bunny who doesn't understand "the horrible truth about the real world."

I've even heard it say that calling on the Power of the Positives is somehow disrespectful for the people who are currently suffering terribly from whatever it may be they are suffering from.

This negative brainwashing about the Power of the Positives is everywhere. It is always a sign that the people who believe this are thoroughly trapped in the fish tank of insanity, on the wrong side of the Energy Chart, without any understanding of our living energy bodies at all.

Without energy, the world becomes hard, crazy, terrifying and all we have to look forward to in life is to grow old and feeble, to feed the worms in the end. This is a horror world, a nightmare and those who believe this are living in hell. Their horizons end at Zero, and through their stress lens, the Positives appear to be some immaterial illusion when in fact, they are the solution.

This leads directly to what I call The Battle for the Positives.

The Positives – POWER, LUCK, LOVE, JOY, ECSTACY, GRACE, HOPE, LIGHTNING, LIGHT to mention but a few! - are not only power-full.

⭐ **The Positives ARE power.**

That is what they are.

They are power for the energy body.

They raise us up on the energy chart and we become stronger, smarter, more creative and far less likely to believe any old nonsense that has been falsely taught by the "authorities of the ages."

Simply put, the bigger and the worse the problem we are dealing with, the more we need that POWER of the Positives to start moving in the right direction to not only solve the problem, but to get to a place where the problem literally implodes and ceases to exist at all.

The Positives are the solutions to problems, they are the absolute inverse of the problems.

I would like you to think of the Positives in terms of hand grenades or nuclear bombs that will take out the problems in an explosion of white light.

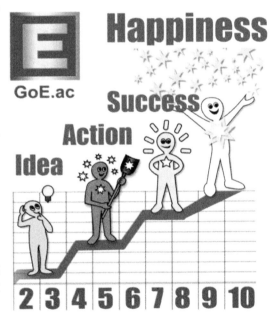

The idea that working with Positive energy makes you weak is simply a great big LIE.

And don't take my word for it. Test it for yourself for a week. Consider what YOU have always needed and wanted, and raise that energy. Find out what happens, and what that does for you.

Start taking back your birthright and experience the Power of the Positives for yourself.

This is reality creation 101.

Positive Thinking

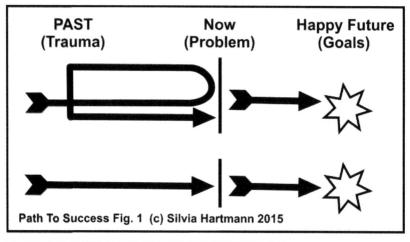

Path To Success Fig. 1 (c) Silvia Hartmann 2015

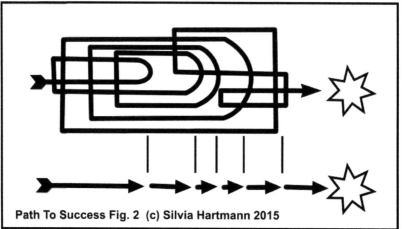

Path To Success Fig. 2 (c) Silvia Hartmann 2015

The fact is that we do not only have real energy bodies, we also have real physical bodies and real physical brains.

When we think the same way all the time, we create train tracks in the brain that take us down the same paths over and over again.

The "trauma brainwashing" has caused people to back flip reflexively whenever there is any kind of problem and created that nightmare labyrinth from which there is no escape.

Any problem that is being encountered causes the brainwashed train track of:

- ➡ I have this problem right here and now
- ➡ This must be so because something went wrong in the past
- ➡ I must find the root
- ➡ What was it?
- ➡ When was it done?
- ➡ Where was it done?
- ➡ Who did it?

Now, we're firmly in a negative energy state, having (yet again) accessed a negative memory and with it, plugged our energy body right here and now, (yet again) into a massive energy drain.

We're lucky if we even remember the problem that caused this time travelling attempt in the first place. We certainly don't think about our goals, our futures.

We have travelled down a train track that takes us in the exact opposite direction of where we actually want to go.

The Artist's Story

There was an artist who had been painting the same picture for 15 years or more. It was a self portrait with a bleeding Christ on the cross forming the eyebrows and the nose. Over time, these paintings became ever more gory, ever more jagged, ever more disturbing.

One day, I came to visit and saw him in his studio, yet again stabbing violently at yet another canvas, painting the picture of his abuse at the hands of a Catholic priest yet again.

I called out to him, "You've been painting the problem for all these years.

"Why don't you paint the solution?"

The artist stopped and turned to me. "But I wouldn't know how to do that. How would I paint the solution?"

I said, "I don't know … if the solution had a colour, what colour would it be?"

He stared at me for a moment, then he cried, "Blue! It would be blue!!!" and he threw the old painting off the easel, got a new canvas, and I left him as he started to paint his solution.

He never painted the old picture again.

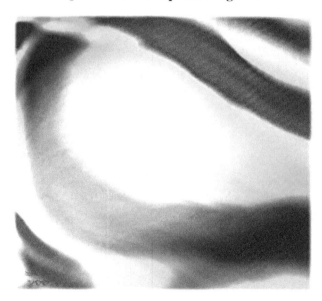

Modern Energy Art Solutions:

Don't paint the problem.

Paint the SOLUTION.

Future Orientation

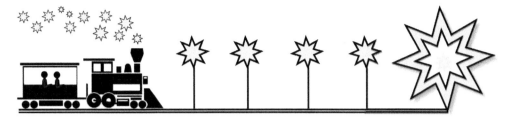

Future Orientation is thinking forwards, rather than back.

- I have this problem that is standing between me and my future.
- What do I need to overcome this problem?
- **WHAT IS THE SOLUTION?**

This is the <u>**direct**</u> path to success.

This is the direction in which we need to think in order to – find the solution!

Re-stating the problem, reporting the problem, whining about the problem, analysing the problem, dissecting the problem and most especially delving into the past to find the trauma root of the problem is not the way forward to a better future!

We need to literally re-train our brains to make new train tracks that will go forward, instead of circling round and round in the fish tank of insanity.

This takes some mental discipline to get started.

It needs for us to become aware that we might be stressed.

That the fact that we are whining, moaning, complaining, doubting, judging, shaming and all the rest is simply an indication that we are energy poor and that we need to STOP.

To take a deep breath.

⭐ **To think towards a positive solution is Positive Thinking.**

We need to replace the old train tracks in the brain with new ones, that lead into the opposite direction.

Towards the new, positive, future orientated direction.

"I am such a failure!" becomes, "What do I need to stop feeling such a failure?"

Well … I might need to experience more SUCCESS, and more frequently!

"What do I need to get more SUCCESS?"

And here we are already on the new train track, the right one, that takes us to a city called SUCCESS instead of that other place, called FAILURE.

- **Our conscious minds have the power to take control of the energy system and turn it this way, or that.**

Thinking towards positive solutions to our (personal, ongoing, daily) problems is a learned, practised skill that gets better, the more we do it.

Aspects Of Love

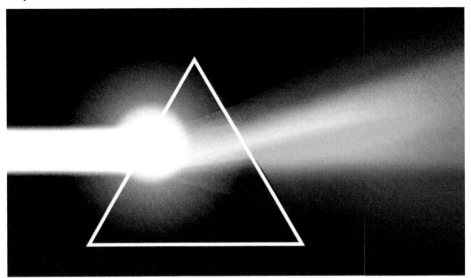

We have to remember that what we call the Positives are all aspects of love.

Love is the most powerful energy in the Universe, and it may well be so that our energy bodies are not ready to deal with that level of power.

That's alright.

We don't need to try and run the most powerful energy in the Universe through our energy bodies just yet.

We can simply start with aspects of love – the Positives, and indeed, the exact right Positives each one of us can feel we need, and hunger for, at any time, and anywhere.

Please note that this is not a Pollyanna approach to ignore problems or avoid dealing with problems.

We need to learn to ask, "What do I need to deal with this problem?" first.

We need to learn to empower ourselves before we delve into whatever problems we need to solve in our lives, because **the solutions we come up with from the stressed states are no solutions at all.**

They are not loving.

They are not logical. Stressed people simply end up creating ever more problems for themselves because they are in no fit state to be making good decisions.

When we are stronger, when we are on the right side of Zero, we start making better and better decisions and at +10, the solutions become revolutionary and truly astonishing.

Working with the aspects of love, the personal Positives, is the right thing to do.

The Healing Solution To The Problem Equation

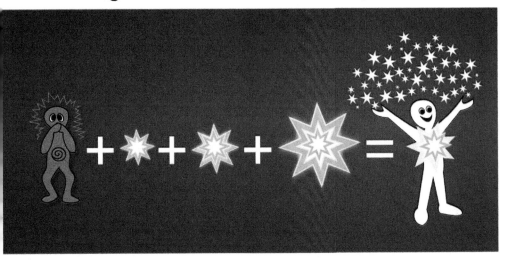

The Positives are the right way to go.

Let me make this very clear.

It is not as though there was a choice between working with Positives, or focusing on the traumas, the old problems and the negatives.

It would be a choice if the outcomes were equal.

This is not so.

We do not arrive at the same place at all.

- **Working with Positives creates a positive outcome, every time.**

It is the right way to go from fear to power, from anger to love, from defeat to victory, from failure to success.

As far as energy is concerned, simply adding the required energy (what we call a Positive) and then the next one, and the one after that, is how to get into higher energy states.

☆ **Keep adding energy, and a threshold shift occurs which transforms the energy body permanently.**

It is simple, logical, correct and entirely predictable.

It is mathematical in its structural simplicity.

In other words, it works.

Expansion And Evolution

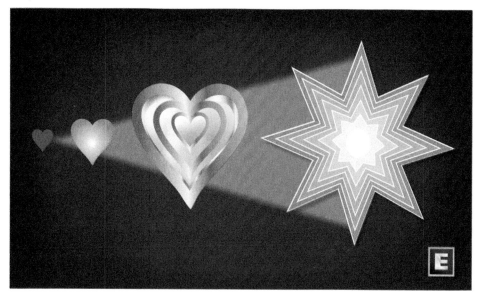

In the same way, as our energy system expands and we enter into the new territory on the positive side of ZERO, our understanding expands.

What was a little red heart that was the symbol of LOVE we go to the Heart of Gold, which expands more and more, until at +10, love becomes a flaring star.

This expansion is the direct effect of the higher energy states.

We understand more, we can handle more power, we have a chance to get to the truth of many things that seemed to be so mysterious.

Above all else, in the higher energy states we have energy enough to start giving, start loving in a whole new way.

Learning How To Love

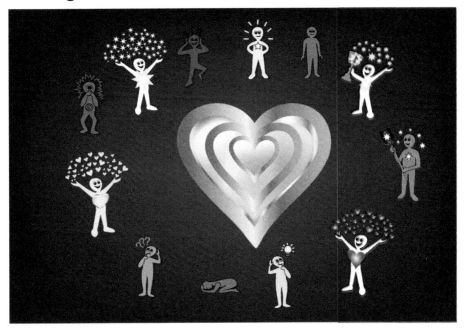

⭐ **You cannot love yourself – but you can learn to love your aspects.**

Love is an outward bound energy. It flows forward, as all things do in the natural Universe and trying to turn it back upon "yourself" causes chaos in the energy body.

Instead of doing that, we can start practising how to love our aspects.

We can start with the easy ones – the successful aspects, the happy aspects who did well.

We can think towards them and receive their energy, and send them our love and admiration in return.

I encourage you to try this; it is one thing to speak of such things in theory, and quite another to have the experience of improved energy flow when you connect with your aspects.

Once you have learned how to do this, you can send Positives to aspects who are still in dire need of energy help across time and space. Let your heart go out to those aspects and give them what they need, then go beyond and into love to raise them and ***transform*** them.

When you are ready, connect with those aspects that you are uncomfortable with or wish had never come into being.

⭐ **All aspects need love to transform.**

The more we practise our loving, the better we become.

The more we have, the more we have to give.

Please understand that our ability to love is not like a bucket that will run out.

Loving in the sense of sending energy to those who need it creates a portal through which more and more love can flow. Eventually, we can love all aspects, even those who are not our own aspects. In loving, we generate the energy we need to have our energy bodies grow up, become strong, become adult, become powerful.

The Starry Future

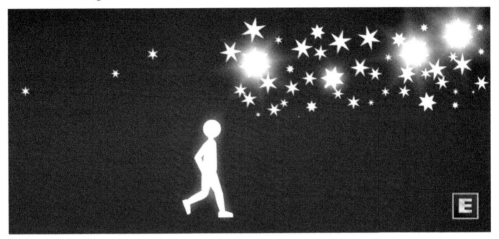

High energy star experiences is what the energy body needs to heal and to evolve.

To have a strong, powerful energy body and experience a different way of life, even if there is no change at all in the strictly material circumstances, we need many, many more positive star experiences.

In the past, these star moments were rare, unpredictable, and deemed to be dependent on money, youth, physical prowess, good looks, being particularly lucky, or relegated to special occasions, such as annual holidays, festivals or getting married.

The older people were getting, the fewer the chances of high positive experiences seemed to become – and nothing could be further from the truth.

- **High positive experiences have always been literally at our own fingertips.**

The Oceans of Energy are all around us – and all we have to do is to make a conscious decision to turn away from the negative, and move forward, towards the power of the Positives.

With simple Modern Energy techniques, we can have a high positive energy experience five times a day.

This will completely transform the way you act, think, feel and behave in under a month.

It soon becomes clear that you don't have to actually "do techniques" all the time to have high positive energy experiences.

Once we unlock the Power of the Positives, we realise that invitations to have high positive energy experiences are all around us, all the time – we were just too stressed to notice.

We didn't know just how much our own happiness matters to everyone.

We didn't think consciously about the importance of adding high energy events to our timelines all the time, every day, every night.

Now we do know. Now, it really is up to us whether we want to take up "The Love Challenge" and start seriously moving into a future that has a thousand times more star experiences than before. This is in our own hands, quite literally.

Plus Ten Is The Only Goal

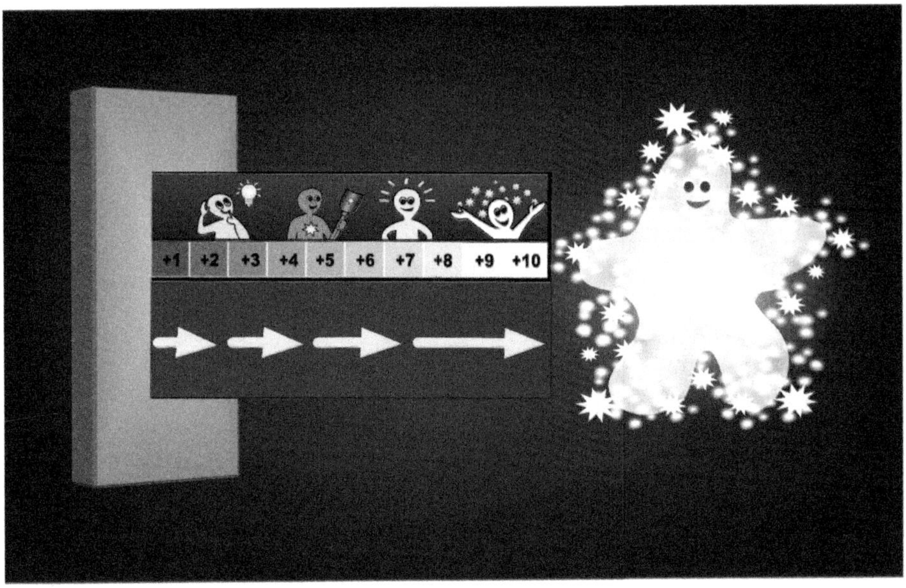

Make it your own personal goal to find out who you really are when you get energy richer, and what happens to your life when you shift your average energy state up by just a few points over time.

Don't be afraid of the many lies that were told about what happens on the positive side of the energy chart.

We don't turn into idiots here who don't understand problems. We don't run around like demented rabbits on steroids, and we don't strip our clothes off and wander the Earth with our rice bowls.

It is true that we don't really know what happens when we get to be higher, but chances are, we are going to be extremely surprised – and amazed, and delighted.

- **With the Power of the Positives, we get to find our own journeys, our own way, each one of us.**
- **We each build our own unfolding path with each step stone of high positive experiences.**

Now that we know this is good, and right, and so very necessary, we can begin our own personal journey of discovery into the unknown world that awaits on the other side of ZERO.

Star Matrix: A New Life

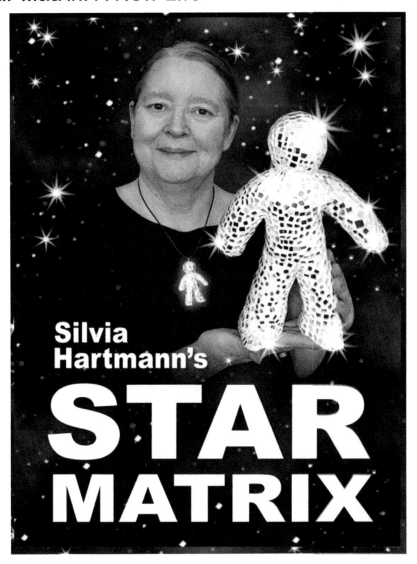

Silvia Hartmann's
STAR MATRIX

"You find yourself at +10."
Silvia Hartmann

There's More To Life Than Trauma!

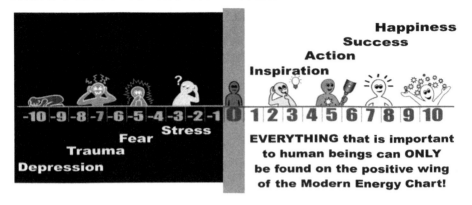

We may wonder why our societies in the Western world are in the sorry states they are in, with all the wonders of technology and so much "progress" being made in so many fields of scientific inquiry.

I would now say that the major reason for the absence of progress as far as human happiness is concerned lies fundamentally in the locked "mind/body duality," and this has produced serious errors and miscalculations. The worst of these is the absolute obsession with trauma, trauma and nothing but trauma.

Trauma events have been the exclusive focus of attention for over 100 years now, and the trauma paradigm is not only deeply entrenched in all human related sciences, it is woven into the very structure of our cultures – in songs, in cartoons, in movies, in novels and the stories we are telling each other, absolutely everywhere.

The fact, or real reality, is that human beings do not only experience more than just trauma, but also, that trauma doesn't actually explain why people do the things they do.

Trauma teaches us what to avoid, what to stay away from, what to fear. Trauma may explain why we DO NOT DO something, but it doesn't explain why we do the things we do.

Trauma teaches us nothing about how to find more happiness, more success in life, who we are, how to go forward – or how to heal trauma.

If we want to learn something about ourselves and each other, we need to stop lying face down in the trauma puddle, raise our head and start looking around what else is really out there.

The Events Matrix

We evolve and change because of energy events in our energy bodies. Energy events create our own unique events matrix, based on our lived experiences up to now. The interplay between our natural progression and the events of our lives form our own unique self. Without taking the reality of the living energy body into consideration, we can never understand what is really happening to us – but when we do, many important insights become revealed.

Trauma

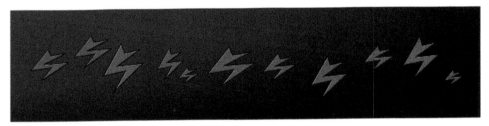

We are in the sorry state at the moment that if we were to ask a person what their life had been so far, they would reflexively immediately think in the direction of trauma. Nowadays, the entire population does this; but it is particularly prevalent among those who have been in therapy.

Unwittingly, they have created for themselves a "trauma matrix" and that is a reality reduced, completely unbalanced and dangerously false model of any human's life.

Guiding Stars

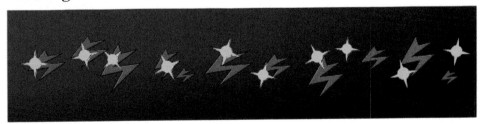

As soon as we had regained the missing positive wing of the Modern Energy Chart, we found a new class of events to explain behaviour – the Guiding Stars, high energy events that did not complete and drive actions to be repeated endlessly.

All philias, addictions, collections and repeating life patterns are not based on trauma, but on Guiding Star events instead: when we add them to the lifeline, it becomes immediately far more interesting, information rich, and we have a new direction for research immediately.

Once we had the two, the trauma spell was broken and we started asking what other kinds of events may be involved in the formation of an individual person in their lives.

Healing Events

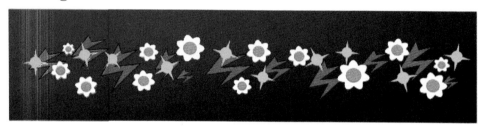

The next type of events were the Healing Events, for example, the wonderful experiences during energy work when a problem not just disappears completely, but leaves the person in a high energy state.

An interesting effect of the Healing Events was that once these had happened, the problem would never come back.

Unknowable Events

We also discovered that people have notable life events which could not be classified as either good or bad.

We called these mysterious events the "Unknowable Events" and added them to the unfolding events matrix.

Missing Events

We also realised that there seemed to be "holes" in our Events Matrix – the Missing Events, experiences that should have been had but did not occur. This continues to be a fascinating avenue of research for Modern Energy.

By adding these different types of actual life events, real lived experiences for real human beings, the lifeline has literally come to life, has started to become far mor interesting, and invites further discussion and investigation.

As if this wasn't wonderful enough already, the most extraordinary threshold shift was yet to come.

The Star Events

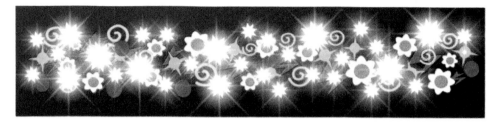

The Star Events are the best moments of our lives.

The Star Events are the precise moments where our aspects achieved the +10 state of being.

Unlike their incomplete neighbours, the Guiding Stars, the true +10 Star Events are complete. They do not need to be repeated, and once they have have occurred, the energy system has evolved and the person is on a new level in their lives.

- **The best energy states, the best experiences of our lives, the most valuable information about you, humanity at large, the universe and everything we could ever know <u>is encoded in those Star Memories.</u>**

The Star Events are also the only type of events that "flashes before our eyes" when we are about to die.

It stands to reason that we should give these Star Memories the attention they so richly deserve.

When we consciously connect with the Star Events of our lives, a fundamentally different as well as profoundly more reality based self concept comes into being, the **Star Matrix**.

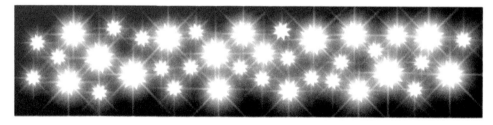

We find the truth of our lives in our Star Events.

Only Love Remains

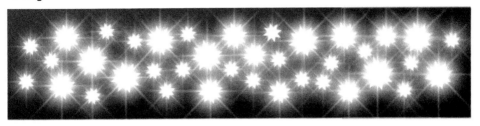

⭐ **The Plus Ten Star Events are the true Treasures & Riches of our lives.**

Memories of our Star Events are the only memories that flash before our eyes when we are about to leave this physical body for the last time.

Only love remains.

We can learn more about Star Events by actively remembering our best positive experiences we have already had. This is particularly important because all of us have been trapped in the fish tank of insanity our entire lives, and we have been brain washed to only remember the traumas, to give the traumas all our undivided attention.

Not only has this been one of the major factors to keep our energy systems down; it has created a totally skewed idea of who we human beings really are. It has further created train tracks in the brain to the degree that some people truly now believe that they never had any good experiences at all.

This is not the case, however. Human beings have the amazing ability to have Star Events even in the most dire of circumstances, and every living person has many, many high positive memories – they simply haven't thought to access them, or understood how important they are.

⭐ **The precious information that teaches us how to have more Star Events can be found in the Star Events we have already experienced.**

When we actively start to direct attention to our own +10 Star Events for a change, wonderful things begin to happen in mind, body and spirit. The quest for the Star Events is the ultimate motivation for all human behaviour.

We are always searching for the next Star.

The Endless Hunger For The Stars

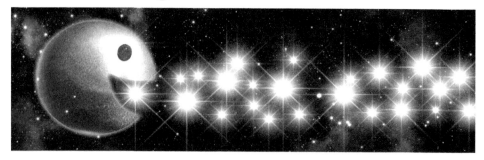

People believe erroneously that they are searching for the next person who will finally make them happy, or for the next object – house, car, private jet, private island; or perhaps they are looking for the adoration of millions who will drown them in applause and money.

- **People are in fact on an endless quest for the next Star Event, the next explosion in the energy body which will evolve them to the next new level.**

The never ending, profound hunger for the next Star Event drives us forward, and once we understand that this is so, we can start to ask completely different questions and find out new paths towards our next Star Event.

Even the simple thought, "I wonder what might be my next Star Event?" frees us from the endless trauma tracks, our own old wrongful conclusions as well as the societally proscribed ideas of what it takes to be happy.

Now, it becomes highly personal and relevant. It becomes interesting.

We can ask further questions. How did other Star Events in my life work? How and where did they occur? In which contexts is it easy and natural FOR ME to experience true Star Events?

⭐ **In order to learn more about these true treasures & riches of our lives, it makes every sense in the world to start by reviewing the Star Events we already know about, our own lived experience.**

Amazingly, when we connect with our own Star Events in consciousness at last, some wonderful things start to happen for mind, body and spirit – and these wonderful things are reality feedback that we are doing something right for a change.

Star Wisdom

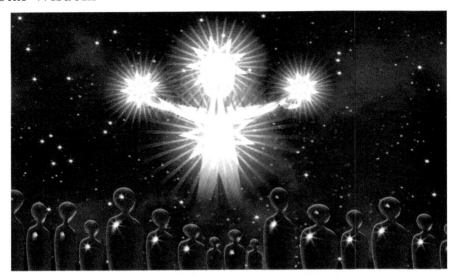

Our own past +10 aspects are "the best versions of ourselves."

When we are in a +10 energy state, we know the most we can know; we understand more than anywhere else on the Modern Energy Chart, and we are the most powerful we can be.

Connecting with our own past aspects who were in very high energy states is infinitely beneficial for mind, body and spirit.

- ★ The energy body is instantly energized when we remember a happy memory.
- ★ The physical body responds also instantly with feeling and functioning better.
- ★ The mind gains access to advanced intelligence, insights and new information.

By connecting with the Star Moments of our own lives, we instantly gain access to energy, power and information which is highly relevant, helpful and beneficial to us, right here and now.

Even better still, by finally starting to pay attention to the Star Events we have already experienced, we are re-focusing our entire system and teaching ourselves not only what really matters in our lives, but also to start to understand how we can have more Star Events in the future.

The Star Matrix

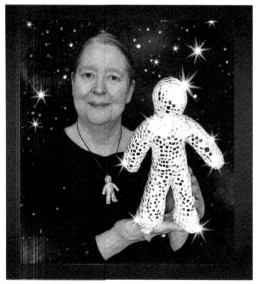

After a lifetime spent trapped in the fish tank of insanity and after a lifetime spent thinking that trauma is all that matters, it is important now to **take an inventory of our Star Events** instead – the true Treasures & Riches of our lives.

When we start to realise that it is truly only our +10 aspects who matter, a different kind of self concept comes into being – instead of defining ourselves by our "scars" we get to define ourselves by our Stars.

⭐ **This creates the Star Matrix – a brand new, sparkling self concept that consists entirely and only of the Star Events of our lives.**

The Star Matrix is not an illusion; it is quite real and comes into being automatically once we have recovered some high positive memories of the +10 events we've already had.

With every Star Event added, the Star Matrix becomes brighter and stronger.

- Our energy systems begin to stabilise.
- We feel more empowered and more protected.
- Our energy average begins to rise.
- The self healing capabilities of mind, body and spirit can finally kick into action.
- Life stops being so hard all the time, becomes easier.

This puts us into a much better position to experience far more Future Stars – of course.

The Star Matrix also provides essential protection and structure for all our systems of mind, body and spirit and helps us to connect with the greatest power in the multiverse at the most personal level – the power of love.

The Logic Of Love

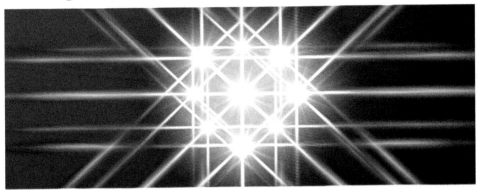

Love really is the one and only greatest power in the Universe.

When we connect with it through personal experience, we are instantly empowered – our energy body becomes empowered, and this lifts our abilities across the board in mind, body and spirit, all together, all at the same time.

There are many things we can do naturally to raise ourselves up by engaging the Power of the Positives and move into that space of wonderment that lies on the positive wing of the Modern Energy Chart.

There are also many, many things we can recognise as being wrong and destructive to the living energy body, and we stop doing those now, and explain to others why we're going to do something else instead.

We can become consciously aware of just how much stress there is in the "world of people" and how all that stress is the direct result of systems that were loveless and inhumane, destructive to human beings in mind, body and spirit.

We can take a stand and say, "I want more than that. I want better than that!"

- **This is the Modern Energy rEvolution.**

It starts by each one of us engaging the drive towards love which is alive in us; it starts by understanding that "our happiness matters" - so, so much more than we have been allowed to understand.

It's all about energy – factoring in the living energy body, and finding ways to empower it, so that each one of us will become stronger, healthier, more intelligent, wiser and most of all, more powerful.

- **Enlightenment is to understand the reality of energy, to have felt it in your own body, and to know that it is real.**

Enlightenment doesn't take some kind of study for decades and it's not about what anyone else has written in some dusty scroll, no matter how long ago it may have been.

We each have our own living energy bodies and we also have experienced the high energy states many times already in the past.

Modern Energy gives us the structure and the thinking tools we need to go ahead and actively now connect with the Power of the Positives, and reap the rewards for so doing all the way in mind, body and spirit.

Modern Energy is simple, immensely practical and entirely built on the logic of love.

It has always waited for us.

It's time now to come home to love.

Everything Works Better With Energy!

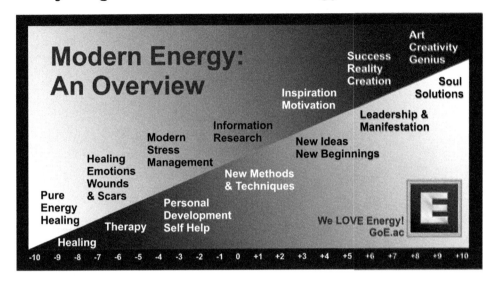

Modern Energy is all about taking the real, living energy body seriously and helping it to heal, to become more empowered, and to evolve.

- When we factor in the living energy body, *everything* changes.

- We can find new ways to solve old problems.

- We can do things differently that are real and have real results.

Above all else, once we step out of the old mindset that keeps humans trapped in the fish tank of insanity on the wrong side of ZERO, we step into a whole new world of possibility, a whole new world where love is no longer just a word.

Our Future Starts NOW!

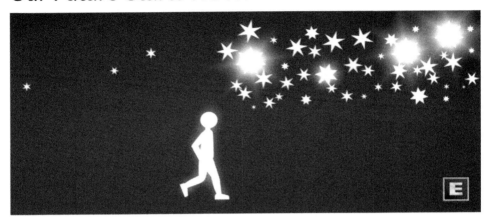

The fish tank of insanity which has trapped people on the wrong side of the Energy Chart is entirely real. It is frightening, overwhelming and absolutely everywhere.

Yet it is an illusion, a misconception created by stressed people over a long time.

To break all of humanity out of the fish tank of insanity is a tall order.

To get one single, individual person to expand their horizons and to start playing with the idea that adding positive experiences to your daily life will make you happier, stronger, more popular, more successful and a better person, that's a different story.

This is where we start.

With me, and with you.

Use your own intelligence, your own experience, and run your own experiments.

Keep the Modern Energy Chart close by and observe the people around you with that additional 16.7% of information that tells you the state of their energy bodies by the way they talk, walk, act, behave.

Pay conscious attention to what happens when you lose energy – what you think, how you feel, how you act, and how others respond to you.

Discover what you are already doing to raise energy, and find out what other ways exist in which you can practically activate The Power of the Positives to raise you up.

Experiment with all the many different energy raising techniques Modern Energy has to offer, and find something that really works for you.

Explore your own Star Memories and connect with your own Star Aspects – and find out what that does for you, right here, right now, in mind, body and spirit.

⭐ Experiment with happiness!

Experiment with your own happiness first of all – what can you do right now to feel happier? Stronger? More glad to be alive? When you are happier, you'll have more to give, and then you can start to experiment with other people.

You can spread a little happiness as you go by … (please try!)

A smile, a kind word, a little bit of FOCUSED ATTENTION in a world where people are stressed, distracted, fractured and isolated is a gift of energy – and it has real, measurable effects that you can see, and hear, and feel.

What happens when you give more energy to this (task, animal, person, situation, group)?

These are the sort of experiments I have been running since 1993, and my experience has convinced me of the reality of energy, of the hard hitting reality of people's living energy bodies and the effects this has on their lives.

Modern Energy is a real, true paradigm shift.

It is a forward movement, a breakthrough in information processing, a door opener to a totally different world – a wonderworld filled with potential, opportunity, and so much more love, fun, joy and personal success than any of us were ever allowed to even dream of.

- **Modern Energy is a rEvolution.**

It's exactly what we've all been waiting for – a sensible way to make sense of being conscious and alive in this life of ours, and to be able to go into the future with great expectations of wondrous things still to come.

Our real, living energy bodies are always striving to grow, to unfold, to expand and to evolve. We start offering even a modicum of assistance to these natural processes that are happening inside each one of us and all the time, and we are rewarded splendidly with new insights, new experiences, new wisdom and more joy in our lives.

The needs of the energy body are simple, and none them require us to be anything other than alive. We don't need to be rich, or young, or pretty, or physically healthy to have amazing energy bodies which will make us strong, glad to be alive, and a real asset to any community or family.

We live in the Oceans of Energy – and our happiness really, really matters!

We need many, many more people who understand that energy is real, and how to make it work for them, so they too can move out of endless confusion, negativity, fear, stress and can help themselves and others.

Join The Modern Energy Revolution!

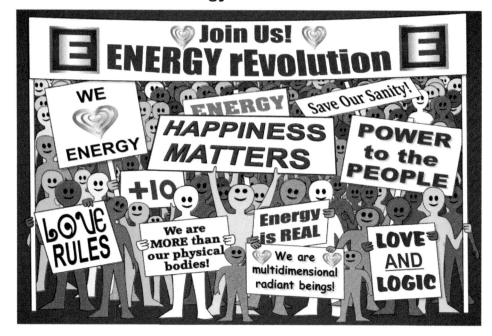

- **I invite you to join the Modern Energy rEvolution today.**

Share the Modern Energy Chart with your friends and family. Simply print it out, put it on the kitchen table and invite a discussion. This simple act literally changes lives for the better!

Share this book with others who need to hear this.

Join the GoE and support us in our work to make the world a happier, more reasonable, more loving place.

It is beyond high time for all of us to make that change from the old five sense paradigm to the new, more inclusive, more realistic one that includes the reality of energy, and to start moving in the right direction, towards love, with all good speed.

Love isn't just a word, or an abstract concept. It is the living energy that created the multiverse, and it's alive within us. It helps us become stronger, wiser, more logical and more loving – all at the same time.

Love is the original miracle. We call it energy – and that's alright for now.

Just know this …

You have an amazing physical body.
You have a beautiful mind.
You have a radiant living energy body.

You are a multi-dimensional being
in the Oceans of Energy -

and <u>YOUR HAPPINESS MATTERS</u>.

I wish you a sparkling fountain of +10 moments to delight you, surprise you, to bring you all those things you've always dreamed of, and beyond.

With all my love to you,

Silvia

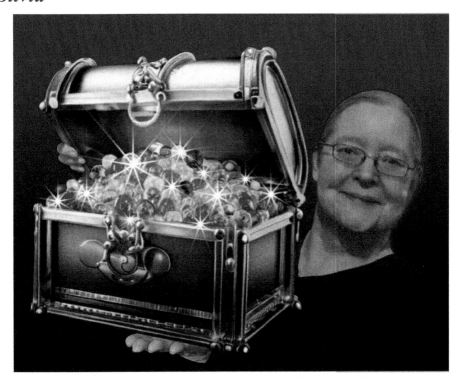

Silvia Hartmann, Creator of Modern Energy
President, The Guild of Energists GoE.ac

Love The Theory? Now Take The ENERGY Course!

Join the Modern Energy rEvolution! Say "NO!" to chronic stress, misery and depression. Discover a treasure chest of wonderfully simple, proven, effective energy raising techniques that are not only loving, but also entirely logical. You can also take an online test and gain your Modern Energy Foundation Certificate. FREE for every GoE Member!

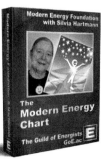
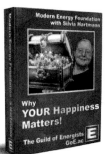
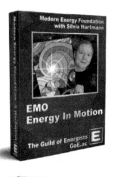
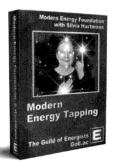
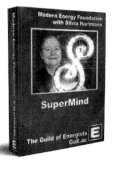
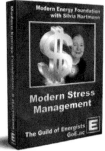
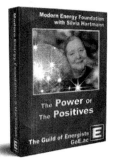
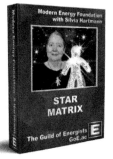

**Join the GoE and start your new, energy richer,
happier and healthier life today!**

GoE.ac/join

About The Guild Of Energists

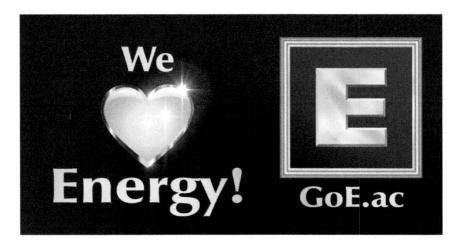

In 1998, Silvia Hartmann created the first Modern Energy organisation to teach the 1st generation of modern energy based techniques which became The Guild of Energists as we know it today.

Modern Energy is The Third Field and Modern Energy professionals specialise in teaching people how to become happier by empowering the real, living human energy body with simple, logical and highly effective Modern Energy Techniques.

The Guild of Energists provides ongoing education, research and inspiration in Modern Energy and welcomes everyone who loves energy to join us in our mission to make people happier!

Modern Energy knowledge is of the essence to help people make sense of their lives, to heal from emotional/energetic wounds and disturbances, to unlock our true human abilities at the high energy states and to provides sound, logical Modern Energy theory as well as effective, beneficial, positive, humane and uplifting practice.

GoE members, practitioners and trainers are transforming the lives of real people worldwide already every day.

Join the Energy rEvolution – join the GoE today!

Further Reading

The Trillion Dollar Stress Solution – Silvia Hartmann

Modern Stress Management

DragonRising.com/Trillion

Modern Energy Tapping – Silvia Hartmann

Start tapping into The Power of the Positives in your life today!

DragonRising.com/MET

EMO Energy In Motion – Silvia Hartmann

The theory and practice of the principles of Modern Energy

DragonRising.com/EMOBook

Star Matrix – Silvia Hartmann

Discover the real and only true Treasures & Riches of YOUR life – and gain a brand new, powerful, protective self concept in the process

DragonRising.com/SMXBook

The Energy of Attraction – Alex Kent

Applying the power of Modern Energy to Love, Dating and Relationships

DragonRising.com/EOA

About The Author

Silvia Hartmann is the creator of Modern Energy and the President of The GoE, The Guild of Energists.

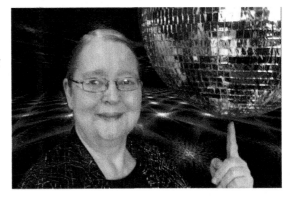

Her original work includes:

1993 The Harmony Program
1996 Project Sanctuary
2000 Guiding Stars
2001 HypnoDreams
2002 EMO Energy In Motion
2003 Art Solutions
2004 Living Energy
2004 Energy Magic
2005 HypnoSolutions
2006 The Genius Symbols
2007 Aromatherapy For Your Soul
2008 Events Psychology
2009 Modern Energy Chart/SUE Scale
2009 The Genius Symbols
2012 Modern Energy Meditation
2013 Modern Stress Management
2014 Modern Energy Healing
2015 Modern Energy Tapping
2016 SuperMind
2017 Modern Energy Art
2018 The Energy rEvolution
2020 Star Matrix
2022 The Power of the Positives
2023 StarLine Therapy

"Love without logic is insanity. And vice versa."

SilviaHartmann.com

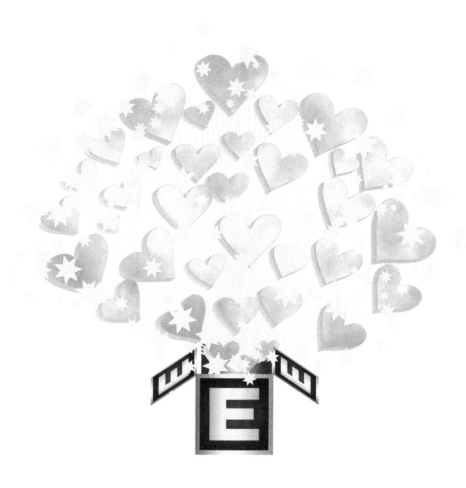

Love this? Join the GoE, take courses and talk to the community:

GoE.ac/Join

Printed in Great Britain
by Amazon

37925125R00076